PRAISE FOR *CHOCK FULL OF NUTS*

"The individual perspective offered in this book is a poignant argument as to why neuropsychiatry must fully transition from a disease-centered model to an individualized, precision-based approach. Treatments must be tailored not just to symptom relief, but also to preserve the person's individuality, function, capacity, purpose, and sense of self. Diagnostic categories are just labels. That requires not just changes in the practice of medicine, but also in the clinical research."

—ALVARO PASCUAL-LEONE, MD, PHD, PROFESSOR OF NEUROLOGY, HARVARD MEDICAL SCHOOL

"JaKob tells the truth in his brilliant portrayal of his frightening incarceration in one of the most esteemed mental institutions. He dares to tell the truth in extraordinary, hair-raising clarity."

—NANCY SCHÖN, AMERICAN SCULPTOR AND AUTHOR

JaKob Williams

MY 28 DAYS INSIDE A

CHOCK

PREMIER PSYCHIATRIC HOSPITAL

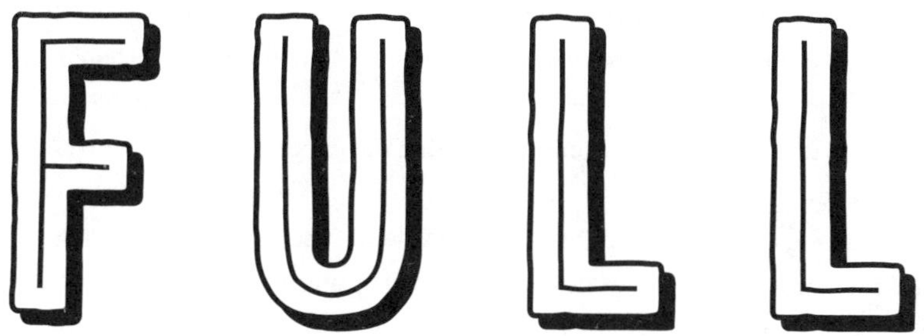

AND THE SHOCKING TRUTH

OF NUTS

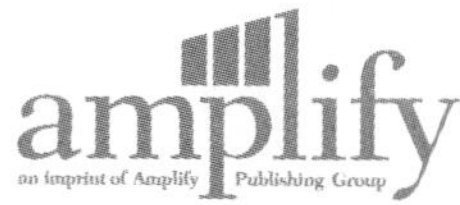

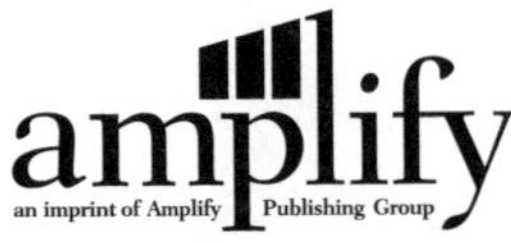

www.amplifypublishinggroup.com

Chock Full of Nuts: My 28 Days Inside a Premier Psychiatric Hospital and the Shocking Truth

Some names, locations, identifying characteristics, and details have been changed to protect the privacy and anonymity of individuals. The author has made every effort to recreate events, locales, and conversations based on his memories. In certain instances, names, occupations, and other identifying characteristics may have been altered or fictionalized to ensure privacy while maintaining the integrity of the narrative. While the author and publisher have taken all possible measures to ensure the accuracy of the information at the time of publication, they do not accept and expressly disclaim any liability for loss, damage, or disruption caused by any errors or omissions, whether resulting from negligence, accident, or other causes. This book is not a substitute for professional medical advice. Readers are encouraged to consult a physician for any health concerns, particularly regarding symptoms that may require diagnosis or medical treatment.

For more information, please contact:
Amplify Publishing, an imprint of Amplify Publishing Group
620 Herndon Parkway, Suite 220
Herndon, VA 20170
info@amplifypublishing.com

Library of Congress Control Number: 2025909214

CPSIA Code: PRV0226A

ISBN-13: 979-8-89138-591-7

Printed in the United States

To Lovely Wife,

Without her, I would not have been here to write this book.

CONTENTS

CHAPTER 1

"IT BEGINS AT CONCEPTION"

When I was presumed dead somewhere on Mount Fuji, I made a deal with either the Good One or the Bad One. If I could live a bit longer, I swore to the Good One to help as many humans as possible, in a bigly way. This book is meant to fulfill that promise as an update to Ken Kesey's 1962 book *One Flew over the Cuckoo's Nest.* Its purpose is to reshape perceptions of mental differences, end some of what I see as inhumane practices, and shine a light on some of the more promising treatments. Yes, I am going to write about the insanity of the existing system to treat the insane. Surprisingly, not much has changed since *Cuckoo's Nest* was hatched. And if my deal was with the Bad One? Well, nothing ventured, nothing gained.

The problem was that when I had the epiphany of my newfound purpose, I was confined to a mental hospital with no good way out. I needed to get out of that place and have it not be the last thing I'd ever do. So, I had to become an exemplary patient, but not so perfect that they'd think I was being manipulative, or worse, "malingering" (psycho speak for lying). I had to maintain focus, avoid electroconvulsive shock treatment (shock treatment or ECT), and wean myself off the heavy-duty drugs. That meant I'd have to abandon my great escape plan, but at least the planning of it would help me eventually write this book.

I frequently reference *One Flew over the Cuckoo's Nest*, which was a significant exposé on the prisons we call mental institutions. My goal is to provide an updated perspective on Kesey's book; I think people will be shocked that so little has changed. While Kesey worked as an orderly in a mental hospital in Menlo Park, California, possessed keen observational skills, and was an excellent narrator, he had one significant handicap—he'd never personally experienced being committed to a psychiatric hospital. I believe that to truly understand another's mental illness, difference, or gift—however you choose to label it—one has to have experienced what the other person has undergone. The "walk a mile in the other person's shoe" idea rings true here.

Too often, I've heard someone try to comfort a friend dying of cancer by saying, "I know what you're going through; my mother died of colon cancer." However, they are more often comforting themselves more than they are the person suffering. No one can truly know how the dying person feels, because the only ones who might fully understand are those who are already dead. A simple "That sucks" might be the better choice.

My advantage is that I've walked the walk and been a player in the big show. I've been committed to the mother of all "Cuckoos' Nests" and inducted into the hall of crazies in the country's first and most prestigious insane asylum, now rebranded MrClean Hospital. I have a debt to pay, and I'm going to pay it. The primary mission of *Chock full of Nuts* will be to shine the spotlight on the supposed "gold standard" for treating severe mental illness, ECT, in the same way that lobotomies were exposed and extinguished in *Cuckoo's Nest*. Regrettably, most people now think that shock treatment has also been discontinued. It is now my job to shock them with the truth.

So, how did I end up in perhaps the world's most famous insane asylum? As it almost always does, it begins at conception. With mental differences, it's all about the genes. My paternal grandfather, Pop, had just graduated from Yale in 1918. Eager to serve as a pilot, he didn't wait for the US Army Air Forces to be officially formed in 1920. He headed to France to join the French Air Force unit Lafayette Escadrille to fight the Germans, who at the time had the most lethal air force in the world.

Pop received his training and dove headfirst into combat. The odds were not in his favor; each mission carried a 10 percent risk of being shot down, which was usually fatal. Now, you might think those odds don't appear that bad. But consider this: Pop flew twenty-five missions, the maximum limit for one tour of duty. When you do the math, the odds of surviving that many missions were a mere 7 percent (0.9^{25}). Given his proficiency in math, Pop was probably aware of the grim odds, especially as he witnessed fellow aviators lose their lives almost daily.

But Pop had no time for discouraging odds. He had his sights on becoming a "flying ace," a coveted title reserved for those who shot down five or more enemy aircraft. At the end of his twenty-five missions, he was only up to three. So, what did he do? He became the first pilot to sign up for a second tour of duty. His superiors couldn't find any rules against it, so up in the air he went for thirteen more. In total, he flew thirty-eight missions over enemy territory and, much to his disappointment, never became a flying ace. However, his stuff was definitely right. Oh, yeah—with the extra missions, his odds of survival dropped to below 2 percent (0.9^{38}).

When he returned from the war, he made a living flying wealthy businessmen from northern Long Island—where *The Great Gatsby* was set—to Wall Street in a seaplane, with pontoons. For entertainment on the return trip in the afternoon, he would fly his clients under the Brooklyn Bridge. Of course, this was strictly forbidden. However, he found a loophole. If the pilot determined that it was necessary to fly under the bridge for safety reasons, he could. Pop made the determination there was a safety issue, almost every day. Eventually the authorities stopped citing him.

Business was good, so he decided to expand and start an actual airline. He secured funding from one of his customers and, after cutting through lots of red tape, received permission to build a ramp near Wall Street. He could literally "fly it to the bank." Unfortunately, a week before his inaugural flight, his investor died of a heart attack. Though another financier client stepped in, when Black Tuesday hit on October 29, 1929, the stock market dropped 25 percent, and the Great Depression began. His potential customers who hadn't jumped off the Brooklyn Bridge were plunged into a Great Depression of their own. His dream of founding the next great airline became a nightmare, and his business folded.

To keep his family afloat, he found work with a banker who had barely survived the crash. The man owned a seaplane and needed a pilot. Although he could only pay Pop just enough to feed his family, lodging was free—a loft in the airplane hangar. After a year or so, Pop got a call from Howard Hughes, who had heard about the daring pilot who'd flown under the Brooklyn Bridge in defiance of the authorities. Hughes invited him to join his team as a test pilot.

Hughes had several radical, untested ideas and needed pilots who were smart enough to understand the new technology and brave enough, maybe even crazy enough, to be the first to test them out. The most revolutionary idea was Hughes's concept that the surface of an airplane should be perfectly smooth. Until that point, engineers thought the rivets used to hold the fuselage together needed to protrude to provide the necessary strength.

Hughes hypothesized that sanding off the rivet heads and making them flush with the fuselage would minimize resistance and maximize lift, allowing for a smaller, more fuel-efficient engine. Hughes had his team of engineers file and sand all the rivets on a prototype airplane until the surface of the fuselage was mirror-like.

On the day of the test run, there was a crowd at Hughes's private airport. He had invited the press and all the employees at Hughes Aircraft Company to witness the event. Most thought it would be a plane wreck. The plane ambled down the tarmac and lifted off just as it ran out of runway. (As it turned out, Pop had done this for dramatic effect, as he could have lifted off halfway down the runway.) Everyone cheered, but the question remained: Could he land it?

On the approach, he tipped both wings and nailed a perfect landing. When he exited the plane, a throng surrounded him. Asked how it felt, he responded that he was just doing his job, and the crowd moved to Hughes.

In 1934, Pop joined the recently formed TWA and rejoined Hughes in 1939 when Hughes purchased the airline. Pop went on to become somewhat of a legend, setting many records for crossing the continent in both the shortest distance and time. He also had to land on a road or two, maybe even a random cornfield; back in those days, planes were not that reliable, and pilots had to continuously look for plan Bs.

He continued as a pilot until his sixtieth birthday in 1956, when the airline notified him that it had instituted a new policy: mandatory retirement at age sixty. After all, how could anyone safely fly a plane after that age? Pop was the first pilot to reach that milestone to fight back.

In a meeting he politely offered, "You guys are idiots. I'm still the best pilot you have. I'm flying."

They countered, "Okay, but you must give up two of your stripes and become a flight engineer."

He left in disgust, called one of his Yale classmates who was one of the country's most distinguished attorneys, sued, and won the case. His settlement was a substantial lump sum payment, which became the template for the first airline pension plan.

Many years later, the asset management firm where I started my career was in competition to manage a portion of the country's largest airline pension fund. There were three firms in contention, and I was the junior member of our team. My job was to carry the booklets and not say a word.

Before the meeting started, the head of the investment committee, a pilot, looked at the cover of the pitch book and asked, "Is one of you related to Pop?"

I raised my hand and nodded.

He walked over, shook my hand, and said, "He was a legend." He then instructed his assistant, "Tell the other candidates to go home; these guys are hired." From that point on, I was allowed to talk in meetings.

So, to recap, Pop was a big risk-taker, had major league self-confidence—bordering on delusions of grandeur—was extremely goal oriented, was a high achiever, believed most people were idiots, and self-medicated with alcohol. I almost forgot to mention, he never slept much. He was pretty much textbook Bipolar II, although he was never diagnosed. If he had been, he would have been labeled a manic depressive back then, a designation first used by the American Psychiatric Association in 1952. (The term bipolar was not officially coined until 1980.)

My dad's story is more succinct. Maxi attended Yale, enlisted in the Army Air Force, and flew a bomber in the Second World War. He joined TWA, then was furloughed twice. He returned to Yale to complete his degree between stints with TWA. He was really smart and thought most people were less so. He self-medicated with alcohol until late in his life, when he started taking Prozac.

Among his eccentric habits were tracking every meal he ate, cataloguing each tomato he harvested, calculating the mileage for every tank of gas, tallying the number of shaves he got from each razor, and keeping a diary of every fishing trip he took—including the quantity and the length and weight of each fish he caught.

But for me, his most memorable quirk was the freezer that shared space in my bedroom. Maxi, being thrifty, would buy food items on sale and freeze them. He didn't worry about the electricity cost since that was included in the rent. Each item was dated, and he used the first in, first out inventory method, ensuring the oldest items were used first. His bread inventory was so extensive that I never ate bread less than a year old, which was pretty unappetizing. He likely had a smorgasbord of mental issues, such as anxiety and obsessive-compulsive disorder, with a side order of bipolar disorder.

So, the odds of my being bipolar were relatively high. Over the last twenty years, I've episodically exhibited many of the symptoms: talkativeness, increased energy, decreased need for sleep, risk-taking, racing thoughts, being wired, excessive confidence, distractibility, increased energy, and agitation. I've found most people, most of the time, to be idiots. The cherry on top? I literally drove Lovely Wife to the brink. At one point more than a decade ago, she warned, "We have a big problem. Either you take meds, or I'll have to, because I'm not sure I can handle this anymore." Guess who ended up taking the meds?

However, it wasn't until the spring of 2018 that the perfect storm hit, when I experienced almost all the symptoms, all at once. So, what was the trigger? In 2017, my college friend Bell invited me to the opening of a major retrospective for Robert Rauschenberg at the Museum of Modern Art (MOMA) in Manhattan.

As I wandered through MOMA, I stumbled upon the centerpiece of the exhibition. It could best be described as "intelligent found art," humbly named *Oracle*, constructed in 1964. *Oracle* is a large, five-part contraption, a fusion of an automobile door on top of a typewriter table, a ventilation duct in a water-filled washtub, a wire basket, a staircase housing batteries and electronic equipment, a wooden window frame supporting another ventilation duct, and five concealed speakers—all mounted on wheels.

What made this seemingly random assembly genius was its ability to simulate the experience of an evening stroll down a New York City residential street on a hot summer evening, circa 1960. Picture this: People would be sitting on their front stoops, smoking cigarettes, sipping their beverages of choice, and tuning into their favorite radio shows. As you walked down the street, snippets of different broadcasts would fade in as you approached and fade out as you moved away.

Oracle couldn't emulate the smoking or drinking part but did a great job on the audio. To create this effect, a team of engineers from Bell Labs had to solve the issue of simultaneously broadcasting multiple AM radio signals. This innovative technology was later adopted by the space program, enabling astronauts to communicate seamlessly with Houston, without a problem.

The masterminds behind this remarkable piece of "art" were Harold Hodges and Robert Rauschenberg. Rauschenberg is well-known for laying the foundation of pop art and found art, but I bet you haven't heard of Harold. Despite having only a high school education, he was extremely curious and had a knack for constructing very complex things. He was a co-inventor of the laser (yes, that laser) and on the team that created the light-emitting diode (LED) found in your TV and everywhere else. So, how did high school–educated Harold end up in the middle of all this?

After serving as a medic in the Korean War, Harold played in a band in the Poconos in northeastern Pennsylvania, famous for its heart-shaped beds. One summer, he met the love of his life. They married quickly and soon welcomed several children. As his band gig wouldn't pay the rent, Harold took a job as a watchmaker—a bit of a misnomer as the main part of the job was watch repair.

One day, a customer came into the shop with a watch he believed to be "probably unsalvageable." Harold smiled and got to work. Within a few hours, he had the timepiece running almost perfectly, deviating by only a few seconds a month from the correct time. This customer recommended Harold to a friend, who told another friend, all with the same results. As it turned out, they were all PhDs working at Bell Labs—named after Alexander Graham Bell. A few days later, an official-looking man in a well-pressed suit walked into the shop.

"Mr. Hodges, I'd like to offer you a job. How would you like to work at Bell Labs as an engineer?"

Harold asked, "How much would I make?" and quickly accepted the offer, which was multiples of what he was making. He realized he had forgotten to ask an important question and followed up: "By the way, what is the job, and who the heck are you?"

Suit-man responded, "Well, I happen to be the head of Bell Labs, and you will be working with about a dozen PhDs. They know the theory but can't make anything actually work."

Harold went on to become something of a legend himself, but was so modest that he would always give credit to the PhDs for his work. He just wanted to have some fun. "They dream it, and I make it come true" was his mantra.

Why is Harold relevant to this story? Harold, it turns out, is the father of Bell, who invited me to the MOMA show. Harold is still alive, in his mid-nineties, and has been totally blind for the last thirty years. He still solves equations on a blackboard with chalk, but only in his mind. When I saw him a few years back, I remarked, "That's pretty old school," to which he quickly added, "That's all they had back then. The tools I use are frozen in time."

After the 2017 show at MOMA, I went to visit Harold. I asked him about his experiences working with the artists. He relayed how hanging out with Warhol and Rauschenberg was a blast. When I asked him which of the group of artists was the most talented, he immediately responded, "Not even close: Rauschenberg. He was an order of magnitude better than the rest."

Harold went on to explain how *Oracle* stayed in his basement for several years "until they could figure out how to simultaneously send and receive multiple radio signals." He added, "*Oracle* was fun, but *9 Evenings* at the Armory in 1966 was 'the cat's pajamas.'"

The *9 Evenings: Theatre and Engineering* performances featured thirty scientists from Bell Labs, including Harold and ten artists, among them Rauschenberg. The two groups collaborated to create art that had never been seen before, incorporating closed-circuit TV, projection TV, infrared

TV cameras, a Doppler sonar device, and Mylar. I asked Harold a question that would change my life: "Which exhibit was your favorite? Which one would you like to recreate?" He quickly responded, "The *Mylar Blimp*. I'd like the *Rising Snowflakes* project repeated as well. Think you can do it?"

I responded, without thinking and in a moment of unwarranted confidence, "Sure."

As I prepared to leave, I asked Harold if he missed not being able to see the seminal art he'd helped create.

He laughed and said, "You don't just see art; you experience art. If all you do is see art, you are missing the point. You must experience art with all five senses—touch, sound, taste, smell, and finally, sight. Art is multidimensional, not just visual. Appreciating art with only 20 percent of your senses is suboptimal. I use 80 percent."

For the next year, I go about trying to recreate two of the exhibits that took ten artists and thirty Bell Labs engineers ten months to complete. How hard could it be? Piece of cake—a thought that psychiatrists would appropriately label a delusion of grandeur. I decide to first work on recreating the *Mylar Blimp* exhibit. Warhol called it the *Silver Pillows*, so I'll use the two names interchangeably.

The *Mylar Blimp*, it turned out, was a zero-buoyancy, pillow-shaped object that appeared to just hover in the air, or achieve homeostasis, as the nerds would say. It created a magical, mystical "Look, Ma, no hands" illusion. Mylar had just been invented by DuPont scientists around the time of the 1966 show.

NASA first used it in 1964 to construct the 130-foot diameter Echo II communication balloon, which was designed to bounce microwaves from one point on Earth to another.

This successful experiment paved the way for today's communication satellites. To increase its versatility, Mylar is layered onto aluminum, which gives it its reflective appearance.

The challenge is how to precisely offset the weight of the Mylar balloon with the lift of the lighter-than-air gas I intend to fill it with. Moreover, the lift has to be achieved at exactly the volume of the Mylar balloon, as Mylar, unlike rubber, does not stretch.

To solve this riddle, I have to solve a set of simultaneous equations with three variables—weight, lift, and volume—and three unknowns. I now understand the overwhelming anxiety that Dorothy, played by Judy Garland in the 1939 film *The Wizard of Oz,* must have felt when she exclaimed, "Lions and tigers and bears, oh my!" If I miscalculate and the lift exceeds the weight, the blimp will rise to the ceiling; if too low, it will sink to the floor. I need the Goldilocks "just right" solution to achieve zero buoyancy. (Nice, I just put Dorothy and Goldilocks together in the same paragraph.)

Time to do the math. No, hold that thought—it's premature. I can't make any calculations until I have an actual Mylar blimp. I also need to decide which lighter-than-air gas to use and where to get it. So, who do you call? Yelp, of course. I search for "industrial gas wholesaler" and find Tolman Manufacturing and Supply, with a perfect 5.0 score and glowing reviews.

Even better, they miraculously have a joke shop that sells party balloons made of . . . Mylar.

At this point, Lovely Wife asks, "Where are you going?"

When I tell her "I'm going to a joke store to buy some helium gas," she gives me a concerned look knowing I'm going off the rails—and not for the first time.

I head there immediately in my "clean" BMW 135i convertible, which in auto speak means there is all kinds of good shit under the hood, but you're not telling. I am greeted by an eccentric-looking, elderly man. I ask to see the owner, and he smirks.

"Go inside. Ask for Brad." Which I do. I approach the guy sitting at a desk behind the counter and ask if I can see Brad.

He laughs and tells me, "You've already met him; he's the guy outside."

As it turns out, Brad is not only a peerless gas guru, but also an adept jokester. His shop is right out of the 1971 movie *Willy Wonka & the Chocolate Factory*. Actually, Brad looks a lot like an older version of Gene Wilder, who starred in the movie. There are five-foot canisters of almost every gas filling the room. I reminisce when I spot the nitrous oxide—used by dentists to knock out their patients and clubbers to get a high. I once tried it at a party thrown by my dentist friend in the 1970s, and it was quite the ride. One puff, and I floated up to the ceiling.

At this point, you might wonder, "Why the hell is this supposedly successful businessman endeavoring to undertake a nearly impossible task in an area, art, for which he has no talent? He must be crazy." Well, yes and no. From my point of view, I have never started a project that I did not finish. I've got balance issues, but I've climbed precarious mountains. This one seems like a small hill to climb.

I gravitate toward the joke section, which houses all sorts of classic joke paraphernalia. This includes the classic palm buzzer—you conceal it in your hand, extend it for a shake, and watch as the unsuspecting target recoils in surprise when the buzzer vibrates. Everyone, except the mark, gets a good laugh. Of course, I buy one on the spot.

Brad approaches at this point, and in a curmudgeonly but playful way says, "You've never been here before. What are you looking for?"

"I'm here to get some advice on lighter-than-air gases," I answer.

"You throwing a party?" Brad inquires.

"Kind of," I respond, and then explain that I need a few Mylar balloons, the biggest he has. He walks behind the counter, grabs two—one a birthday balloon and one a bachelorette balloon—and comments, "These Mylar balloons can stay inflated for a whole week. The rubber ones deflate in about twelve hours."

I good-naturedly respond, "I'll take the bachelorette party ones; I've been hired as the entertainment." I quickly add, "The reason the Mylar balloon stays inflated is because the helium atoms are larger than the pores in the Mylar, thus keeping it inflated. On the other hand, the helium atoms are smaller than the rubber pores, so they leach through, causing the balloon to go soft."

He steps back and with a wry grin asks, "What the hell are you really up to?"

I explain that I'm working on recreating a 1966 show created by a bunch of scientists and artists who experimented with gases, and that I heard he knew something about gas.

He says, "Maybe. What do you have in mind?"

I give him three words: "Zero buoyancy, homeostasis."

He halts, stares at me with a gleam in his eye, and announces, "I'm in. I've been wanting to solve the zero-buoyancy problem for years. Why the hell didn't you start with that? I knew no bachelorette party would hire you. Let's get to work."

I ask, "When?" and he commands, "Now."

Brad tells his guys that he'll be busy for a while, and I proceed to cover the details of the Mylar blimp project. My goal is to find a gas that's lighter than air to counterbalance the weight of the Mylar balloon, enabling it to hover in midair. I postulate that mixing two gases with different atomic weights might be more effective, as this would let us regulate the lift of the gas within the Mylar balloon's fixed volume by varying the proportions of the two gases. I'm thinking about using nitrogen (N_2), with an atomic weight of 28, and helium (He_2), with an atomic weight of 4, both of which are lighter than air, which has an atomic weight of 29.

Brad replies, "That is exactly the right approach, but there's some good news and bad news. The good news: There's plenty of nitrogen, as it makes up 80 percent of the atmosphere."

"What's the bad news?" I ask.

The bad news: "Helium is almost impossible to get your hands on. It makes up a minuscule fraction of a percent of the atmosphere. It can be extracted from the earth's crust, similar to natural gas, as it is a byproduct of radioactive decay. However, that is expensive. Even worse, we're in the midst of a housing boom, and blowtorches used in construction consume vast quantities of helium. Likewise, surging demand for computer chips, where liquid helium is used to cool the magnets involved in chip manufacturing, has made the shortage worse."

"So, no can do?" I ask.

He quickly counters, "I said 'almost impossible.' I'll get as much as we need."

On my way out, he hands me a big box filled with heavy-duty gas gauges, a gas mixer, a coil of three-eighth-inch id (interior diameter, for the layperson), vinyl tubing, and two heavy five-foot canisters of gas—helium and nitrogen.

He also offers some advice: "Forget trying to crack the equations; focus on solving the problem. Use trial and error."

Of course, why didn't I think of that? The *Silver Pillows* (Mylar Blimp) project now seems achievable, and with Brad on board, I have a great addition to the team.

However, there is still a long way to go. The *Rising Snowflakes* puzzle will be even more difficult. As Harold and his daughter explained it, a column of bubbles arises from a Chock full o'Nuts coffee can and continues rising in an unbroken stream for ten feet or more. Each column would consist of over a thousand bubbles, filled with lighter-than-air gas, each bubble connected to its neighbor. Ah, there lies the connection—both projects require lighter-than-air gases that fill a space encompassed by heavier-than-air material: Mylar for the blimp, soap for the rising snowflakes. However, soap bubbles are much trickier than Mylar.

Getting *Rising Snowflakes* right might be difficult, but a pot of gold awaits if I succeed.

The effect is magical: The glistening bubbles look like snowflakes. However, they turn gravity on its head, rising rather than falling. When light strikes the bubbles, they emit a spectrum of dazzling rainbow colors, represented by the acronym ROYGBIV: red, orange, yellow, green, blue, indigo, and violet. This effect hasn't been replicated since the *9 Evenings* at the Armory show over a half a century ago. At this juncture, I can't help but wonder if I've ventured too far "over the rainbow," I'm "balancing on a tightrope" without a net, or I'm simply "in over my head"—pick your favorite cliché. Just then, my phone vibrates. It's Harold's daughter, Bell, inviting my motley crew to the Poconos in Pennsylvania.

They've discovered an old prototype of the Chock full o'Nuts can used in the original *Rising Snowflakes* exhibit at the Armory, along with some of the hardware. It was literally gathering dust in their basement. *Road trip* is the first thought that pops into my mind. I feel a weight lifting off my head, which gives me the idea for the perfect title for our show, *Defying Gravity*. After all, that's the essence of our project.

Bell says we can come up any time, so I propose, "How about tomorrow?"

She enthusiastically agrees: "Let's do it."

I immediately recruit two eager companions for the drive to the

Poconos, because every road trip needs company. Thelma took Louise, although, come to think of it, that didn't end so well. My sidekicks are a well-respected SoHo gallerist, Georges Bergès (GB), who has agreed to assist in the staging of the newly christened *Defying Gravity* show, and a former celebrity columnist for *Vanity Fair*, George Wayne (GW). He is renowned for his acerbic wit, provocative queries, and penchant for referring to people who meet his strict standards as "Darlinka." In other words, the perfect road trip companion.

I let Lovely Wife know the plan, and she gives me the usual "Good luck with that" before I hop into my BMW 135i convertible and head for New York City. The convertible only holds two, so on the way I order a sedan for the trip and decide to splurge on one night at the One Hotel, a block below Central Park.

The next day, I go for a run in the park, then head to the Hertz counter a block away from the One to pick up my rental car. I've reserved a Prius, wanting to appear environmentally hip. They tell me that they do not have a Prius available. Instead, they offer me a Toyota Corolla.

I laugh and reply, "Don't insult me; I ordered a Prius, and I want a Prius."

Their retort: "How about a premium, convertible Mustang?"

"No, I want a Prius," I insist.

"Perhaps an Escalade?" they smugly offer.

I counter, "A Tesla would be acceptable," wanting to seem reasonable, and knowing that Teslas are even hipper with the green crowd.

No luck. I then reveal that I am directing a documentary film titled *Weird Harold*, about the most creative and prolific scientist of this era. I tell them if they help me, I will include them in the documentary. Immediately, they pick up the phone, call the central office, and hang up smiling.

They say, "How about a Maserati SUV? Six hundred horsepower, zero to sixty in four seconds, a top speed of one hundred seventy-five, brand new, fifteen miles on the odometer, and . . . for the *same* price as the Prius."

I respond incredulously, "Maserati doesn't make an SUV; they would never stoop that low."

At that moment, a blue Maserati SUV emerges from around the corner, purring like a kitten but capable of roaring like a lion. They hand me the keys, and I'm off. I drive to the gallery to pick up GB and GW.

They glance at the Maserati, then at each other, and exclaim in unison, "How the hell did you get that?"

I reply, "I really wanted a Prius, but I guess this will have to do."

Off we go, through the Holland Tunnel into—wait for it—New Jersey.

Despite having a GPS, I get hopelessly lost in Newark. We fall behind schedule, but no worries—I have a Maserati, baby. Approaching a red light with both lanes backed up for a quarter mile, I head down the breakdown lane. I hate people who do that, but sometimes you got to do what you got to do. When the light changes, I floor it. Everyone's head snaps back, and soon I see only tiny specks of cars in the rearview mirror.

We reach the Poconos in record time, and Harold and his daughter are there waiting at their off-the-grid house by a lake—no street number, no street name, only polar coordinates to find them. We have a nice lunch, go for a dip in the lake (one of us sans suit), and then hear Bell yell, "Lunch is ready!" We head back to the house. As we open the refrigerator to put the mustard back, Harold mentions that it goes on the second shelf from the top, two inches from the left wall and two inches from the front.

Although totally blind, Harold has memorized every square millimeter of the house. If the mustard is not placed precisely there, he won't be using it for a while, and he is particularly fond of mustard. Bell then hands me a bag filled with a potpourri: a Chock full o'Nuts can, assorted tubes and connectors, and some soap bubble solution.

I look perplexed, but she just says, "You'll figure it out. Now get out of here—time for Harold's nap."

We hear Frank Sinatra singing "Fly Me to the Moon" as we depart.

The return trip is mostly uneventful except for a pit stop in the bowels of Newark, where once again I lose my way. GW signals that he needs to "take a pee." I pull over near a telephone pole where several locals are hanging out near a lot filled with junk. GW prances over to the pole, unzips his fly, and "takes a pee," then jumps back into the car with his usual impish grin. I should add that GW is sporting one of his typically stylish, flamboyant outfits, complete with bare midriff. The locals try to appear unimpressed. He grins at them and says, "Bitches, *that's* why they call it a junkyard."

After dropping GB and GW off at GB's gallery, I head uptown back to the One. I hand the keys to the valet, who looks in awe at my wheels. It's early evening, and as I'm strolling through the lobby, I notice an interesting group—black men, a few Rastafarians, and a couple of corporate types—all glancing around nervously.

Attired in my usual all-black outfit, complete with black hat, black-rimmed glasses, and black Prada sneakers, I'm waved frantically over.

They ask, "You the damn Uber driver? Where the hell have you been?"

I tell them I'm not, but then I pause a minute and think, *Why not?* So, I tell them, "Actually, I'm Lyft, Lux Black XL. Where to?"

They introduce themselves as Toots and the Maytals, and they need to get to the Jimmy Fallon show in ten minutes, as they are the guest musical performers. For those not familiar with reggae music, Toots is a Jamaican legend, on par with Bob Marley. My Maserati is still parked directly in front of the hotel on Fifty-Eighth Street. (They leave the sweet rides outside to impress the impressionable.) We all pile in, and I take off fast, really fast, like hitting sixty in four seconds fast. I turn onto Fifth Avenue, and head for 30 Rock, where the Fallon show is filmed. I cover the mile in less than a minute.

Whether or not I ran a few red lights is irrelevant; the important thing is that I got them there on time.

As they're getting out, one of the business types says, "We owe you big time. Come to Jamaica, and we'll show you a good time."

One of the Rastafarians chimes in, "Hey, mon, we own the largest ganja farm in Jamaica. You can take as much as you can carry." They make the show and are dope.

In the morning, I return the Maserati to Hertz and thank them for the car.

As I'm leaving, one of the guys calls out, "Don't forget us in your movie."

I reply, "You guys will be the stars," and they all smile. I walk over to my BMW and drive back to Boston with Harold's box.

Once home, I take the box to my workbench and open it to find an eclectic mix of items. Most important is the Chock full o'Nuts can. I'm surprised to also see a bottle of Jack and Jill Soap, no doubt for the bubbles. However, I decide to literally shelve the *Rising Snowflakes* project for a while. It has many moving parts, and it's starting to induce what I can only describe as high anxiety—an allusion, of course, to Mel Brooks's classic 1977 film.

Ticktock—the clock is ticking. We visited Harold in April of 2018, and I have a deadline of September 5, which not coincidentally happens to be the thirty-ninth birthday of Lovely Wife. To be accurate, it will be the twenty-seventh celebration of her thirty-ninth birthday, but who's counting? So, 150 days to go.

Time to get to the hard work. Surveying the garage, I decide to start with getting the silver pillows to float. Brad has supplied me with dozens of "naked" Mylar balloons. As a major customer, he was able to get the supplier for his joke shop to give us balloons with no printing on them. After all, this is a serious art show—so "Bachelorette Babes" emblazoned on my pieces wasn't going to fly, no matter how tempting.

I study the gas hardware and figure that Brad must have given me all the parts I need. Like a jigsaw puzzle, I just have to put the pieces together in the right way—how hard can it be? After a week of fiddling and diddling—an expression made famous by Boston Celtics radio announcer Johnny Most—I am fairly sure I have it figured out.

A few days later, I still can't fill the damn Mylar balloon. My self-respect doesn't allow me to ask Brad for help. It took me a day to finally see the little flat indent that opens into the balloon when pushed. You insert the tube, turn on the gas, and ideally the balloon inflates. But in my case, the standard plastic tubing doesn't fit correctly, and the balloon inflates and then . . . collapses. After a dozen or so attempts with the same result, I remember Einstein's definition of insanity: "doing the same thing over and over again and expecting a different result."

Undeterred, I take a break and drive to my favorite ice cream stand, Dairy Happy, and order their most excellent root beer float. They get a 4.1 on Google with 437 reviews, but a lower 3.0 on Yelp with 235 reviews. They get dinged on Yelp for mediocre $29.95 fried clam bellies—as they should. The root beer float arrives with a silver aluminum straw with about a 30° bend in it. I look carefully, and it appears to be the exact shape and size I need to inflate the balloons.

I rush home, put the root beer float in the freezer for later consumption, and head to the garage. One end of the straw fits perfectly into the polyethylene hose. I take the proverbial deep breath and insert the other end into the balloon, step back, turn on the gas, inflate the balloon, take out the straw, and—wait for it—see a perfectly inflated balloon that immediately rises to the ceiling. Too much lift. I now heed Einstein's advice of not repeating the same failed experiment and begin to vary the proportions of the nitrogen and helium gases to find the Goldilocks solution. (As an aside, I've always wanted to put Einstein and Goldilocks in the same sentence.) Employing trial and error with the gas ratios, I am unable to get the balloon to hover in mid-air. It either rises to the ceiling or falls to the floor, with an 80 percent nitrogen–20 percent helium ratio as close as I can get.

Frustrated, I take the inflated balloon upstairs into our living room for a change of venue and let it go. It goes up a little, down a little, and eventually stabilizes in midair. I rush to tell Lovely Wife—who couldn't care less—and the Mylar balloon follows me at waist level.

The question perplexing me is, "Why does the balloon float in mid-air in the house, but not in the garage?"

Just then, Lovely Wife chimes in. "Did you remember to turn the AC on? It's getting warm in here."

"Yes," I reply curtly.

Suddenly, the answer hits me: Unlike the house, the garage is neither heated nor air-conditioned, with the temperature remaining pretty consistent from floor to ceiling. However, when the AC is on in the house, it creates a significant temperature differential—at least five degrees—from floor to ceiling.

I consider the physics at play here. The balloon rises until it hits the warmer, less dense air, which provides less lift. This causes it to drift lower until the cooler, denser air nudges it back up. Over time, the balloon reaches an equilibrium and hovers in mid-air, achieving zero buoyancy.

This reminds me of how a pendulum works: When you pull the weight out, it swings with ever-decreasing amplitude until it comes to a stop. I drive over to tell Brad, and he is kind of excited: "Wow, zero buoyancy."

When I realize that I am the second one to achieve zero buoyancy in this manner since the 1966 Armory show, "I feel good" (James Brown, 1964). The first was the Warhol Museum in Pittsburgh, which showcases *Silver Pillows* as their centerpiece featuring around twenty-five Mylar balloons floating in mid-air. I vividly recall them years ago during a visit to my son, who was attending Carnegie Mellon University, and we stopped by the museum. Our tour guide mentioned that it was Warhol's favorite exhibit. If you get a chance to visit, look out for the plaque with Warhol giving credit to—wait for it—Harold for creating it. I'm in good company.

I can already hear some of you geeky weather conspiracy theorists out there bitching, "You are so wrong about that!" Okay, weather and spy balloons operate on the same principle, but they can't float in a living room. More succinctly, my response: "Get a life."

I make yet another trip to SoHo to meet with GB to work on the plans for the September 5 event. He claims to have located a fantastic space in Chelsea, large enough to handle the crowd we're expecting, and with a ceiling high enough to accommodate the rising columns of bubbles. It also boasts an intriguing feature, a large curved white wall, the ones advertising agencies use for supermodel photo shoots. Hmmm.

Following dinner, I head to Washington Square Park, always a happening place. Street musicians, jugglers, kids blowing giant bubbles, others running through the fountain, intense chess matches, dogs running in the dog park, picnickers on the grass, and people smoking and selling grass. But today I observe an additional attraction: a piano situated near the arch, complete with pianist and a large crowd gathered around it.

I ask a guy with a red checker piece in his earlobe, as in checkers the board game, "What up?"

He replies, "It's piano night. They have it whenever Colin feels like bringing his piano."

I glance over just as a tall, good-looking guy—more like an Adonis—hops onto the piano and belts out "Largo al factótum" in a powerful baritone. You know the tune—it's the one with the repeating "Figaro, Figaro, Figaro" from *The Barber of Seville*. Suddenly, a crowd forms as hundreds of people run toward the piano from every direction. Pure magic is happening; they hear the voice, see the face, check out the body, and are in love. When he finishes, there is not a sound. No one moves, except for me.

I head to the piano just as the crowd erupts in waves of "Bravo! Bravo! Bravo!" His name is Emmett.

I tell him, "I'd like you to sing at an event, on September 5. It's to pay homage to the 1966 *9 Evenings* show at the Armory, perhaps the most important art event of the century."

His immediate response: "I'm in."

I ask him, "How much do you usually charge?"

Emmett replies, "Normally, seven thousand dollars plus a thousand dollars for the piano player. But for this event, I'll do it for free . . . if I can bring my mom."

"Deal."

Emmett will be singing in front of the large, curved wall in the Chelsea event space with its serendipitously excellent acoustics. The theme of the evening is defying gravity, after all. What better way to get the crowd aroused than Emmett? He'll be one more transcendent part of the evening's events; those curved walls will be vibrating.

With the ladies . . . with the gentlemen . . .
Everyone asks me, everyone wants me, women, children, old people, young ones:
Here are the wigs . . .
A quick shave of the beard . . .
Here are the leeches for bleeding . . .
Figaro! Figaro! Figaro!

"Figaro," *The Barber of Seville*,
Gioachino Rossini, 1816

Back to Boston, and I begin to realize the enormity of what lies ahead. There is going to be a major art event, with press coverage, high expectations, and way too many moving parts. GB, in his typical understated way, posts on his website, "It's going to be the event of the year, not to be missed." For hyperbolic gems like this I only half-jokingly refer to GB as "P. T. Barnum 2.0."

As expected, the riddle of the soap bubbles, a.k.a. *Rising Snowflakes*, proves to be much trickier to solve than the Mylar blimp puzzle. Each column of bubbles in *Rising Snowflakes* contains numerous individual bubbles, all connected to their neighbors. What invisible hand is holding them together? The simple answer: surface tension.

The more complete explanation? The lower surface tension of the detergent in the soap solution allows a soap film to separate from the surface of the solution, forming a perfect sphere. This is the bubble's preferred shape, as it maximizes the ratio of volume to surface area. Furthermore, bubbles will group together and share some of their surface area, as this further reduces total surface area, increasing the ratio further. This is the physics—and the magic—behind the beautiful column of *Rising Snowflakes*. Once again, Lovely Wife drifts through my workshop and sees me surrounded by copper tubing, gas tanks, and a Chock full o'Nuts coffee can, singing, "I'm gonna take you higher" (Sly and the Family Stone, 1971). Once again, she looks concerned, knowing if I go much higher, it won't end well.

The easy part is getting the bubbles to rise. Injecting pure helium gas into the soap solution causes the column to rise way too quickly. The rapid ascent overpowers the surface tension that holds the bubbles together, causing the column to break apart, with just fragments floating to the ceiling.

On the other hand, using regular air causes the bubbles to rise too slowly, and the column collapses on itself. How to adjust the speed of ascent? Easy, use the Mylar blimp playbook: a mix of helium and nitrogen. For *Rising Snowflakes*, I figure a small dose of helium will suffice—less than what was needed for *Silver Pillows*, given that soap film weighs far less than Mylar.

To test this hypothesis, I bring back my new best friend, trial and error. A blend of 90 percent nitrogen and 10 percent helium does the trick, the trick being a beautiful column of bubbles rising at just the right speed to maintain integrity while ascending in a straight line. I won't delve into how frustrating it was to find the proper soap solution. Who knew adding glycerin for the proper viscosity was so crucial? On the hardware side, Harold's prototype was a huge help; all I had to do was attach the polyethylene tubing, without straw, to the original Chock full o'Nuts can. Without that, it would have been, "Chelsea, we have a huge problem."

CHAPTER 2

"WIZARDS EXIST, AND I'M HARRY F'ING POTTER"

It is now the end of June, and the big event—the recreation of the *9 Evenings'* thirty-ninth birthday extravaganza—is just sixty-five days away. The wheels on the bus are going round and round and picking up speed. I'm pretty sure at this point Lovely Wife believes the wheels are going to fly off.

The days fly by. The Silver Pillows are mostly finished, and a proof of concept for the *Rising Snowflakes* is complete, but there's still a long way to go to get it ready for prime time. Since I aim to outdo the Armory exhibit with three columns of bubbles, I need to find two more vintage Chock full o'Nuts cans and trick them out with all the necessary hardware. A jingle comes to mind: "Chock full o'Nuts is the heavenly coffee." Right now, it's more like hell.

At that moment, I have an epiphany. Why did the artists and engineers use that specific brand of coffee can? Duh, it was a triple entendre: a brand name for coffee, it describes male genitalia, and they were all *nuts*. It made sense. The artists were nuts, but the engineers? Most were from MIT, and I recall overhearing a conversation between two women at a party: one married to an MIT engineer, the other in search of a suitable mate. The married one shared sage advice with her friend: "At MIT, for a woman, the odds are good, but the goods are odd." Odd, peculiar, off-center, nuts, so yeah, the MIT crowd belonged.

I extend my working hours to 18/7, or 126 hours a week. Eight hours at my day job, and ten on *Defying Gravity.* Four hours of sleep a night maximum. Instead of feeling exhausted, I wake up full of energy and hot to go. Sometimes I go to bed grappling with a problem and wake up with the solution. I become increasingly agitated. To me, everyone except for the people on the *Defying Gravity* team is an idiot. I start to drive extremely fast, between home, job, and SoHo.

After all, I have a souped-up custom BMW 135i convertible that goes zero to sixty in under five seconds, with a top speed of close to 180 when the governor is disabled, so why not use its full potential? I don't think my driving is unsafe. From my perspective, everything appears to slow down when I'm driving fast, my reflexes are quick, and other cars seem to be barely moving. I can see far ahead and plot my optimal path as I weave through the traffic.

Wayne Gretzky reportedly experienced a similar phenomenon on the ice. I *am* Wayne Gretzky. I start to talk exceptionally fast, or, from my perspective, everyone else talks very slowwwwly. My spending becomes excessive, at least according to Lovely Wife. I tell her I'm investing, not consuming—there's a difference. I am easily distracted and tell the same story over and over, the same story over and over, did I mention that I tell the same story over and over?

Just about then, I come to realize my true purpose, something for which I have been groomed since birth. My history now makes sense. After all, why did I have the only perfect score ever on the IQ test, in fourth grade? Yes, they gave IQ tests to children in the 1950s and then "tracked" them. I should add that it was "technically" a perfect score. IQ tests are multiple-choice and begin with the easiest questions first. I got the first eight questions right: B, C, A, D, | B, C, A, D. I saw the repeating pattern, filled out the remaining answers in the same order, and handed in the test after just ten minutes, to a perplexed-looking teacher.

She asked, "Are you feeling sick?"

I responded, "No, I'm finished."

About six weeks later, my mom got a call from the principal, who wanted to discuss something with her, and to bring me along. I got really scared. I knew what this was about. Maybe I'd been wrong about the pattern and scored really, really low on the test, or I'd been right about the pattern and scored so high they thought I was a cheater. Either way, I was in trouble.

In the conference room, the principal and two serious-looking men in suits—who said they worked for a testing company—were waiting for us.

Just as one of the test guys was informing my mom, "Your son is a genius," I blurted, "I cheated."

They were taken aback. "How did you cheat?"

"I saw a pattern and just went with it."

They looked at each other in disbelief. "That is impossible. We have a team of some of the best statisticians in the country to ensure every test is meticulously checked and double-checked for integrity."

I explained, "I saw a pattern in the first eight answers: B, C, A, D | B, C, A, D, and I just filled in the rest that way."

My principal interjected, "Very clever. You gentlemen should check that out."

To their horror and chagrin, they did check it out and found that I was indeed correct. For good measure, they threw out my score.

Apparently, the designers of this test were tasked with making the answers random. Their interpretation of randomness, which was wrong, was an equal number of each letter choice. The easiest way to ensure this was the "repeating letter shortcut." Just as most people think that the coin toss sequence H, T, H, T, H, T, H, T, H, T is random, or 50/50, it actually isn't. However, it does have an equal number of heads and tails. The actual probability of that sequence being random is less than one out of a thousand, specifically $1/2^{10}$ or one out of 1024. But who's counting? The brain trust at the IQ test company applied the same shortcut, using B, C, A, D repeatedly. It could have been worse—they could have gone with A, B, C, D.

Now it all becomes clear. That test maker was a lazy idiot, and I was the only one clever enough to ferret him out. I am smart. I am better than everyone else. Having just had cataract surgery, lost weight, and upgraded my wardrobe, it's obvious that I AM THE CHOSEN ONE TO

LEAD THE EXISTENTIAL BATTLE OF GOOD VERSUS EVIL. This is a quintessential delusion of grandeur, the essence of mania, but to me, it is all true. Instantly, my brain sifts through the various saviors. Am I the ancient Ma'at, the Egyptian who fought the evil Isfet, sower of chaos and disorder? No, I kind of like chaos. Jesus Christ, who sought to save souls? No, I dress better. Neo from *The Matrix*? Getting closer, and with Carrie Anne Moss playing Trinity, who's hot in a kick-ass way, it's not a bad choice. No, I am a different "One": I am Harry Potter. Harry Fucking Potter. This recreation of the 1966 Armory show is just a ruse, a thought planted in my mind by—wait for it—Dumbledore. Harold is the mastermind. He is Dumbledore.

Wizards exist, both good and evil, along with a multitude of Muggles. I categorize people first into Wizards and Muggles, and then sort the Wizards into good and evil. It turns out that it's easy. Wizards have a distinctive look: Their eyes reveal that they possess special powers. Also, this is a quintessential case of "It takes one to know one." For the good versus evil part, since I don't have a sorting hat, I'll use my gut.

I realize that the good wizards are already all around me. My family and friends have been waiting for me to come to that realization on my own. The cast of characters includes Dumbledore/Harold; Hermione/Lovely Wife; Ron/my friend Barry; Hagrid/my business partner Ernie; Defense Against the Dark Arts Professor Remus Lupin/my MIT professor friend Jay; Luna Lovegood/my daughter; and rounding out the cast, Fred and George Weasley/my two sons.

Most importantly, I have the two best protectors one could ask for. My Bernese mountain dog, Matilda, is the perfect Fluffy, guarding our house and family fearlessly. She is freakishly fast and strong for her breed. Second, Moai, a sixteen-thousand-pound exact replica of an Easter Island moai head, made from pink granite. She is indestructible and incredibly powerful, facing south because that's the direction from which the bad things come.

One might ask, what is a sixteen-thousand-pound moai head doing in my backyard? Of course, it makes perfect sense. There was to be a total eclipse of the sun on July 11, 2010. I've always wanted to see a total eclipse, make that *dreamed* of seeing one. It just so happened that Easter

Island was the optimal place to view it, with over four minutes of totality. That is the moment when the moon completely blocks the sun, revealing the elusive corona. I had been denied my dream of seeing an eclipse earlier in life because "eclipse glasses," which you use to look directly at the sun, were not available.

Back in the 1960s, conventional wisdom held that even a fleeting glance at a partial eclipse would blind you, as any portion of the sun was so intensely bright it would melt your retinas. Rather than directly looking at the sun, you made a box with a pinhole and a piece of white paper on the opposite side of the box. By sticking your head into the box from the open bottom, you could see the light entering the box through the pinhole and a bright dot appearing on the opposite side. This dot would gradually reveal the eclipse's progress, with a dark shadow in the shape of a crescent—the moon's silhouette passing over the sun.

However, the box thing was not very satisfying. Much like having sex in a rubber suit, it might be happening, but you aren't really feeling it.

In addition to being the perfect location to witness the eclipse, the island is famous for its mysterious moai heads. Carved from volcanic rock, they originally encircled a large portion of the island, all mysteriously facing inward. They were huge, some over thirty feet high and weighing more than seventy-five tons. Nobody knows what they symbolized or how the Rapa Nui, the island's residents, moved them from the inland quarries to the coast.

They accomplished this roughly a thousand years ago, without the benefit of a Caterpillar backhoe, draft animals, or even—wait for it—wheels. Their culture had not yet discovered the wheel. How the hell did they do it? It literally took the whole village. They stood the moai up on end and tied three ropes around the statue—one on each side, and one in front. A group of five or six Rapa Nui would grab each rope. The group on each side would rock the moai, and the ones in front would pull forward. This is called walking the moai. It took a long time, but it got the job done.

The moai cannot be removed from the island, even for a billion dollars. However, twelve have been pilfered. Chile possesses three, France has three, the UK and the US have two each, and Belgium and New Zealand each have one. The Rapa Nui, using moral suasion, are aggressively trying to retrieve them. They are currently in intense negotiations with the British Museum and the country of Chile. For the Rapa Nui, retrieval is nonnegotiable—they have been looted, much like the Jews who had their art looted by the Nazis during World War II.

The Museum of Natural History in New York City badly wanted a moai but failed to get their hands on one. Instead, they made a replica. The museum made it, not out of clay, but even worse, fiberglass. This replica is featured in the 2006 movie *Midnight at the Museum*, starring Ben Stiller.

Serendipitously, both the eclipse and visiting the moai on Easter Island were near the top of my bucket list—a one-two punch too tempting to pass up. I immediately and gleefully went about figuring out how to make it happen. Lovely Wife, who claims she does not have a bucket list—arguing that only immature men do—agreed to tag along.

Getting to Easter Island was not going to be easy. Even though the eclipse was a year out, apparently there were other "bucket listers" competing for the few airline tickets and hotel rooms needed for the stay on Easter Island. Eventually, I found a high-end travel company, Abercrombie & Kent, which claimed to have "just a few spots available," for a mere $25,000 per person—meals not included.

I was ready to go for it but decided to do a little due diligence first. What was the typical weather that time of year? Bad news: Weather.com said, "The probability of cloud cover is greater than 50 percent." FIFTY percent. If there were a 50 percent chance of divorce, would you still get married? Okay, that was a bad example. But, if there were a 50 percent chance that you would lose a $50,000 investment, would you go for it? Probably not.

I moped around for a while before a solution hit me. I wouldn't go to Easter Island. Instead, I would get my own moai head. Not a chintzy fiberglass one, nor an actual one made of volcanic rock and likely to disintegrate in a few centuries by acid rain, but one that would be standing for more than a hundred million years. I had heard of a quarry in Chennai, India, that still had pink granite available and local craftsmen who would carve the granite into any desired shape.

It would take two men one year to carve it, but the upside was that they would each work for a dollar a day. You read that right: one dollar a day. I emailed them specifying that I wanted a moai head and attached pictures of the one I liked from the Museum of Natural History. I offered to pay the craftsmen two dollars a day. They immediately responded in the affirmative, provided wire instructions, and requested payment in full.

They couldn't wait to start. Periodically, they sent me pictures showing the progress, with the craftsmen standing in front of the moai, with wide, mostly toothless smiles. The task involved cutting a block of the pink granite, lifting it out of the quarry, and then using a hammer and chisel to hack away at the granite block. The finished product looked perfect.

Michelangelo is said to have described creating the statue of *David* as simply removing the excess marble; *David* had always been there, and all he had to do was reveal him. I had two Michelangelos, and they had freed Pink Moai from the block of granite that had imprisoned her for hundreds of millions of years.

No doubt, like the genie being released from the bottle, forever grateful moai would diligently protect my family from all danger. Just one overlooked problem: How to transport pink moai to her final destination in a suburb of Boston? The Chennai craftsmen had to wait for the end of rainy season, so that the muddy roads would be firm enough to move her. From there, it was on to the loading docks of Chennai, into a container, onto a cargo ship. Then travel ten thousand miles via the Indian Ocean, through the Suez Canal, across the Mediterranean and the Atlantic Ocean, to Newark. From there, she went onto a tractor-trailer to the end of our driveway. A three-foot deep hole was dug in our backyard—it had to be deeper than the frost line—and filled with crushed stones. Then, an enormous Caterpillar lifted her up and placed moai on top of the stones. It's exhausting just writing that.

As for the eclipse, another total eclipse was to occur on August 21, 2017. This time, it would be visible from the top of one of the Grand Teton mountains in Wyoming, where there was a 90 percent chance of a clear view. I booked it immediately.

Moai is powerful, but she is a protector, a defender, not a weapon. If you are going to defeat evil, you can't just play defense. In chess, playing defense, at best, results in a draw. You only win if the opponent is stupid. Evil isn't stupid, and a draw isn't good enough. Evil must be defeated. I need a weapon, the most powerful weapon ever made.

At this point my brain lights up, literally, I can feel the synapses firing on all cylinders.

What is the opposite of defying gravity? It's gravity itself. I had seen the beauty of soap bubbles floating up, forming perfect spheres. I now have to flip the math. Because the sphere is the most efficient shape to maximize the ratio between the volume and the surface area, it is also the most compact way to store mass. My weapon will consist of a very heavy sphere, the most efficient way to pack a punch.

This is where Sir Isaac Newton comes into the story. He is the father of all things gravity and the namesake of my favorite childhood toy, Newton's Cradle. For those who had a deprived childhood, a Newton's Cradle is a device that simply and brilliantly demonstrates Newton's laws of motion, using balls: perfectly spherical, nickel-coated, chrome steel balls.

It is composed of five such balls hanging closely together in a line from a metal "cradle." They swing freely, attached to the cradle with monofilament fishing line. You pull one ball out and let it go. It then hits the other four balls with a clink, causing one ball to shoot out the other side. The launched ball then joins the other motionless three balls. The ball that shot out then reaches its apex and swings back down, and the process continues for a long while. If you pull out two balls and release them, then two balls pop out the other side while the two launched balls remain still along with the middle ball. The middle ball never moves. The other two balls continue their trajectory.

The real magic happens when you pull out three balls and let them fly: Not only do the two end balls shoot out the other side, but the first of the three balls that makes contact keeps on moving with the other two, and just two balls remain behind. This goes on not just once, but ten or twenty times until all the balls eventually come to a stop.

If you slept through your physics class, or worse, did not take one, a quick review is in order. Newton's three laws are: 1) The law of inertia: A body at rest stays at rest, and a body in motion stays in motion. 2) The law of acceleration: The acceleration of an object is positively correlated with the net force applied and inversely proportional to its mass. 3) The law of action: For every action there is an equal and opposite reaction.

All three are seen in Newton's cradle. For the nerds who never got a high school prom date, maybe me, the reason the balls don't go on indefinitely is due to friction, such as the weight of the fishing line, air resistance, and so on. However, Newton's cradle is just a toy, albeit a great one. I have been chosen to lead the existential war of good versus evil. This is no ordinary fight; this will determine whether humanity survives, or pure evil reigns. Evil already lords over hell, and it must be stopped before it also claims Earth. To do this, I need to create the most powerful weapon ever: the world's largest Newton's cradle.

Since the balls will be doing the heavy lifting, I name the project *Newton's Balls*. The first step is to make a prototype as proof of concept. I quickly sketch a likely candidate and decide to begin with the frame. I'm off to Home Depot and go straight to the plumbing section. I grab fifty feet of one-inch threaded pipe of assorted lengths and a box of threaded elbows and rush home. Miraculously, I manage to fit the segments of pipe into something resembling my sketch.

On to the balls. Determining the optimal diameter of the balls is posing a problem. I decide to search the internet for "balls." Unfortunately, the porn filter is turned off, so male genitalia fill the screen, not that there is anything wrong with that. Why didn't I do the search in "private" mode? Lovely Wife periodically uses my computer and "inadvertently" looks at my search history, and that search would be "hard" to explain.

Eventually, I stumble upon the website of Dick's Sporting Goods. Just a fifteen-minute drive, and appropriately named for this project. They have massage balls in four-inch, six-inch, eight-inch, and ten-inch sizes, and I head for them immediately. They need to feel just right in my hands.

Lovely Wife sees me heading to the car and asks what's up. I inform her that I'm going to Dick's to fondle some balls. Once again, I can see she doesn't understand the importance of my mission. She looks very concerned, and I see her grab her phone and start frantically dialing. After an hour of fondling, I find that the six-inch ball is too small, lacking the wow factor.

The ten-inch ball is too big, too much to handle. But the eight-inch ball is, as Goldilocks would have said, just right. By this point, I've attracted a bit of a crowd wondering what the hell I'm doing.

Undeterred, I proceed to the next stage of ball selection. The massage balls provide the right size, but I need kinetic action, and they don't have it. A vision pops into my head of Pelé, the legendary Brazilian soccer player, kicking a ball over his head, facing away from the goal, into the net. His average of a goal per game is unmatched. That's it—soccer balls are the answer. I run to the soccer area of Dick's and discover that the Junior Soccer League balls have the exact eight-inch diameter I'm after. I purchase five.

The final piece of the puzzle: finding the right string to attach the balls to the frame.

Monofilament line, typically used by anglers to connect the hook to the reel, should do the job. Monofilament line is used by fisher-people to attach the hook to the reel. I jog over to the fishing section, searching the shelves until I locate twenty-pound test line, which should be strong enough to handle a moving soccer ball yet light enough to have little effect on the momentum.

Monofilament is hard to work with. However, my many years of fishing with my fishing fanatic father have prepared me for this. We used to wake up at 3:00 a.m. to reach Barnegat Bay early enough to cast our lines at dawn, when the fishing is the best. Tying these knots will be a piece of chocolate molten cake.

Back in the garage, I need to find an effective way to attach the line to the balls.

Borrowing from the silver straw playbook, I realize a straw is, once again, the solution. One more trip to Dairy Happy, one more root beer float, yields me one more straw. Back to my shop, I cut the straw into five pieces. With the help of our reliable Gorilla Super Glue, the metal straw segments are firmly attached to the top of the balls in seconds. The rest is easy: For each ball, I thread the line through the metal straw and attach each end to the top bar of the frame, using a perfection knot. The balls are spaced a little more than eight inches apart—slightly wider than the diameter of each ball.

I call Lovely Wife over, and she begins filming with her iPhone as I pull back one of the outside soccer balls, then let it fly. It collides with the other four, and the one at the opposite end shoots out, exactly as Newton predicted. Next, I pull two balls and then three, and they behave exactly as expected.

"HUZZAH!" I yell. I loved the streaming Hulu series *The Great*. Elle Fanning was superhot as Katherine, and when she shouted that word in the great hall, every man would stand erect. Now it's time to transform the prototype into the world's most powerful weapon: *Newton's Balls*.

The hardest part will be obtaining the metal balls. They need to be metal, because the Newton's cradle toy uses solid metal balls for a reason, and I want to be as true to the original as possible. Metal possesses the best kinetic properties. I figure that ball bearings are the way to go, given they are made from chrome steel and are perfectly spherical. The diameter is within a thousandth of an inch in any dimension, just as perfect as a soap bubble.

However, how to find an eight-inch chrome steel ball bearing? Once again, I turn to my intelligent friend, Google. I query "eight-inch chrome steel ball bearings." I get back one-eighth-, three-eighth-, up to seven-eighth-inch ball bearings. I try again, "jumbo chrome steel ball bearings," and an intriguing response pops up: "Giantnewtonscradle.com." Huzzah, once again. I click on the link and, holy shit, find some guy, Zach, based in Florida, who sells Newton's cradles—with four-inch nickel-coated chrome steel balls—for $2,395.95.

I immediately hop on the phone and contact him forthwith; you must admit that sounds classier than "right away."

I inquire about Zach's background. He has a day job, but his passion is building Newton's cradles. He makes the biggest in the world, and while sales are slow, his real return is the pure joy of making something he loves and selling them to people who love them back.

I ask, "What are the biggest nickel-coated chrome steel ball bearings you can buy, and why the nickel coating?"

He answers, "Six inches."

Despite the low-hanging fruit, I don't bite on this one. He continues, "Nickel plated because it gives you a mirror finish, and the reflection surpasses da Vinci's glass globes."

My kind of guy—he knows da Vinci well.

I ask, "Just curious, how many days a month do you get five hours of sleep or less, and how often do you think someone is an idiot?"

He replies, "I never get more than five hours, and I think someone is an idiot all the time. Don't you?"

Combined with his rapid, excited speech, it's not hard to see he probably has a good case of hypomania—a bonus for the job ahead. He's a fellow member of the club.

I know about this club because Lovely Wife informed me of my membership in it about a week ago.

I asked her, "What's hypomania?"

She told me to Google it. Yep, that's me. I search on and find a study reporting that a disproportionate share of the CEOs of the S&P 500 companies, most of the top lawyers, scientists, academics, doctors, artists—you name it—are hypomanic, or its big brother, manic. But there's a dark side to it; the successful ones are just the tip of the iceberg. Many end up homeless, in jail, or in an insane asylum, which they tactfully call a "mental health facility," where they join others who suffer from depression, psychosis, and schizophrenia, among other maladies.

Now for the big question: "Can you get your hands on eight-inch nickel-coated chrome steel ball bearings?"

Zach replies, "No one has ever manufactured one."

Disappointed, I ask, "So, it's not possible?"

Zach answers, "I didn't say not possible. I've dreamed of this my entire adult life. It's the perfect size. Let's go for it." And off he goes, a modern-day Knight of the Round Table on a quest for the Holy Grail.

For the next two weeks, we text constantly—noon, midnight, three in the morning, it doesn't matter. I go from five hours of sleep a night to four. Zach literally searches the world and the seven seas. He first approaches the US manufacturer who makes his four-inch balls.

Their response: "No fucking way anyone can make them."

He scours the internet and finds three companies that make "military-grade chrome steel ball bearings."

He contacts them all—one in Germany, one in Sweden, and one

in China. The Germans and Swedes tell him six inches is the largest they have ever made, and in their expert opinion, that was the theoretical limit. In other words, "No fucking way." That translates in both German and Swedish to "Auf keener fall" and "Inget jävla sätt," for completeness.

They assert that a single flaw in the ball bearing could make it explode upon impact with another ball bearing, which could kill someone.

The Chinese company doesn't respond, leaving me dejected. I guess six inches will have to do, but it is a big downer. Like thinking you're marrying a princess and waking up to discover she is Phyllis Diller. Just then, Zach gets an unexpected call. A guy named Kan Dew introduces himself as the manager of the ball bearing plant in Chongqing—the most populous city in the world with over thirty million people. Dew claims he can manufacture the ball bearings.

Zach figures there has to be a translation error. "That's 20.32 centimeters."

Dew responds, "Yes, I understand. I have my PhD from MIT. I can manufacture the balls. It will be very hard. The minimum order will be fifteen balls, and it will cost fifty thousand dollars."

Zach says, "Hold on," and calls my cell.

I say, "Hell, yes. Just don't tell Lovely Wife."

For the mental health professionals out there, you know excessive spending is another symptom of hypomania. But, just to be fair, this was spending the appropriate amount for making history.

The good news is that in addition to being an expert on balls, Zach is also proficient at attaching the balls to a cradle. He immediately orders galvanized steel aircraft cable with "relatively high tensile strength." To allow room for error, he chooses cables capable of holding a thousand pounds. Now, we just have to wait for delivery, expected in a month. Given that it is early July, the balls should arrive by early August—assuming they arrive at all. With the event scheduled for September 5, I'm in deep shit. I begin working twenty-one hours a day, morphing into what Lovely Wife accurately refers to as "Hulk mode."

I decide to drop by my office—after all, I'm supposed to be the CEO.

As soon as I walk in, one of my partners, the chairman of the board, grabs me and points to a conference room.

He says, "I've been talking to your Lovely Wife, and we agree that you need help, though we know you won't accept it. Other people in the office only know that you're working on an art show in New York City. It is obvious that there is something 'off' with you, even more off than usual, so I'm telling you to not to come back to the office until this is resolved. I'll cover for you."

I incredulously ask, "Will I still get paid?"

The chairman replies, "Not only will you get paid, but we'll give you an extra $1,000 for each day you stay away from the office."

Resigned, I mutter, "Okay," and head home.

Now it's time to take inventory. So, what needs to be done? Well, pretty much everything.

I immediately start searching for a stainless-steel fabricator to construct the frame for Newton's Balls. I also need to allocate some time to fine-tune *Silver Pillows*. On the other hand, *Rising Snowflakes* requires significant work, particularly since I've decided to go with three *Rising Snowflakes* stations for a better wow factor—as well as two-up Harold. I do need help.

I drive to see Brad and ask him for a recommendation for a stainless-steel fabricator in the area. He points across the street.

"Smith & Sons, ask for Paul—he's the best in the business."

I head right over. It's an all-business business with a large American flag on display as you enter. I follow the sign to the office and see the business manager, Stan, through the glass door, who waves me in. Fortunately, I look the part, wearing a T-shirt, blue jeans, and steel-tipped black work boots. More importantly, I've made my hands filthy by rubbing them over a greasy generator at Brad's. I know places like this don't like soft-handed college boys. I had a summer job in a shop like this and got ruthlessly hazed. Instead of trying to explain what I need to Stan, I ask for Paul directly.

"Paul who?" he responds.

I know this trick, the runaround, so I respond, "Paul, the guy old man Tolman told me to see. By the way, he says you're still a lousy poker player."

He laughs and points across a large airplane hangar-like warehouse filled with all sorts of steel fabrication jobs, all manned—yes, all men—with huge muscles, dirty T-shirts, jeans, and steel-tipped black boots. "Over there, near the back to the left," he directs.

The workshop looks something straight from Occam's razor, which states that you should solve a problem in the most direct way, with the fewest number of steps. William of Occam was a fourteenth-century philosopher who gave us the principle of parsimony.

The guys here can fabricate just about anything and do it in the most simple but elegant way—in other words, no bullshit. Best of all, I have the crème de la crème, Paul. He seems straight out of central casting: a big, friendly head, crooked-toothed smile, messy hair haphazardly arranged, muscled arms, and hands like the Hulk.

When I reach out to shake his hand, I realize that his viselike grip is likely to turn my hand into pulp, but I give it my best shot and manage to not grimace upon contact. As I begin to explain the *Newton's Balls* project and mention the eight-inch chrome steel balls part, he stops me.

"No one has ever made eight-inch steel balls—I know steel balls," he smirks. He probably has steel balls. He continues, "It can't be done. They'd weigh about eighty pounds, and could be dangerous if flawed. That's why nobody's tried."

I ask him how he knew so much about chrome steel balls, and he points to a stack of math and physics books and says he is working on a master's in physics at night, but don't tell any of the guys, or they will rag on him.

"If I can get my hands on them, can you fabricate the cradle part?" I ask.

"Hell, yes. I'd love to do it. Just give me a sketch, and I'll make sure it gets done in time. However, I'll need the balls in my hands to finish the job—and it won't be cheap," he responds.

I query, "How not cheap?"

He parries, "Fifty grand."

As I turn to go, I tell him, "Okay, just don't tell Lovely Wife," and bid him . . . adieu.

Now the shit is hitting the fan. My punch list consists of:

1. Acquire two more Chock full o'Nuts cans for the *Rising Snowflakes* exhibit, bend the copper tubing into a circular shape to place at the bottom of the cans, drill holes in them, and attach plastic connectors so I can attach the gas.

2. Get four helium tanks, sixty pounds each, and four nitrogen tanks, a little heavier, since nitrogen is heavier than helium.

3. Buy two more gas mixers, really expensive copper gadgets that combined two gases into one, $1,500 each.

4. Confirm Emmett, the opera singer, and assure him that the venue has the required acoustics, and check the ceiling heights for *Rising Snowflakes.*

5. Write the PR piece explaining what the hell we are doing; GB, the gallery guy, will post it to his hundred thousand Instagram followers and blast it out to his ten-thousand-strong email list.

6. Get my hands on the balls, get the sketch for the *Newton's Ball's* cradle to Paul, and have the balls, if they ever get made, and wires, shipped to his fabrication facility.

7. Have Zach and Paul coordinate with each other on the balls, arrange to have the Newton's *Balls* disassembled, driven to SoHo, then reassembled in GB's gallery.

8. Plan for Zach and Paul to have hotel rooms near the gallery, etc., etc., etc. Oh, I forgot: one more huge lift.

9. Lovely Wife suggests that we recreate the scene where Marilyn Monroe's dress gets blown up while standing over a subway grate as a train passes below; she thinks it is the perfect defying-gravity moment. I quickly agree, believing it is both a most excellent idea, with the fringe benefit of distracting her from the cost of the project. Little did she know that her plastic surgery budget is blown, and she'll have to look her age.

Where to begin? I decide to multitask, as there isn't enough time to do just one thing at a time. There is NO time for sleep now, just twenty minutes of meditation a day, lying on the floor wherever I happen to be: GB Gallery, an outside park bench, you get the idea. Now I really understand what the term "24/7" means, and suddenly the Korean convenience store on Thompson and Prince in SoHo and I have something in common.

Miraculously, I manage to complete one through five on the list, even writing the PR piece. The balls are put on hold for now; they're too heavy a lift for me now. So, on to number nine: recreating Marilyn's famous subway grate scene. It raised her acting profile as much as it raised her dress. I Google "Marilyn Monroe subway dress."

As I'm becoming increasingly agitated and distracted, I ruminate about Google's name.

The spelling is blasphemous. Any novice mathematician knows the proper spelling is googol, representing 10^100, or 1 followed by 100 zeros. The largest known named number. Okay, MIT geeks, there is a googolplex, a googol to the googol power, and you might as well throw in infinity as well.

The search result reads, "On September 15, 1954, Marilyn Monroe's iconic scene for the movie *The Seven Year Itch* was shot on the southwest corner of 52nd Street and Lexington Avenue; her then husband, Joe DiMaggio, was apoplectic." I'll be heading there soon.

Further down the search page, a Quora question catches my eye: "Was Marilyn Monroe a sapiosexual?" I can't resist, so I click on the link: "Probably, yes." I then Google "sapiosexual," and to my great delight discover that a sapiosexual is someone who wants to have sex with a genius. It goes on to say that Marilyn once confided in a friend about her desire to have sex with Albert Einstein. Now that would have been a big bang.

I hop into the BMW and head back to SoHo, checking into the SIXTY SoHo Hotel. The next morning, I visit the gallery and brief GB on the concept for the Marilyn exhibit, and that I'm planning on using the actual subway grate from the movie.

He questions somewhat skeptically, "How are you going to steal a subway grate at one of the busiest corners in New York City?"

I reassure him that it's a piece of cake; I'll create a diversion to clear the police out of the area.

He responds, "I don't want to know."

I have a few hours to kill before the mission to "acquire" the Marilyn subway grate, and another "ingenious" idea comes to mind. My balls are designed to be the ideal size for someone to grasp one, pull it back, and then release. Many of the tricks will require a person on each end. For some reason, it makes sense to me to hire two women named Hannah for the role—ball puller.

Hannah is a palindrome, which reads the same backward as forward, much like the backward and forward motion of my balls. Hannah, my favorite Peloton instructor, is serendipitously scheduled to teach a live class in the Peloton New York City studio soon. I reserve a place, arrive early, spot Hannah, and approach her to inquire if she'd be interested in the role of a ball puller. Not surprisingly, two security guards apprehend me and escort me off the premises.

Oh, well. Time to grab the subway grates. I punch the location into Google Maps, and it instructs me to take the Lexington Avenue subway uptown, get off at Fifty-First Street, walk one block north, and stand on the southwest corner. I inspect the subway grates and find the one featured in the publicity poster for the film for which Marilyn posed. I'm armed with a crowbar to pry it up, not as suspicious looking as you might assume—after all, who doesn't carry a crowbar on the New York City subways?

I'm attired in my usual "caper outfit": nondescript black hat, black balaclava covering part of my face, a basic black long-sleeve shirt, black jeans, black gloves, and black socks. For wheels, I'm wearing black Converse sneakers; everyone in New York City wears black Converse sneakers. I try to pry up the grate, but it's been soldered shut. Evidently, other obsessive Marilyn fans have tried the same. Somewhat dejected, I measure the grate and come up with a plan B.

The next morning, I drop by the gallery before heading home.

GB is pacing the floor nervously and asks, "Did you do it? Did you do it? I can't believe you did it."

I'm perplexed and ask, "Do WHAT?"

"Blow up the whole fucking city block! There was a huge steam pipe explosion last night. Every emergency vehicle in Manhattan was there."

I pause for a moment, "Did anyone die?"

"Holy shit, you did do it," he groans in disbelief.

"GB, I'm not saying I did or I didn't. If I admit to it, it will confirm your worst fears. If I deny it, you will think I'm a liar." I just tell him that the Marilyn exhibit is a go, and people will just have to wonder about the origin of the subway grate, including him.

He ends with, "I don't want to know. I need plausible deniability."

I bid him . . . adieu and head back to Boston.

The next day, I call the New York City Transit Authority and ask them about their subway grate supplier. They transfer me to the construction department, where the operator connects me to Joe. He asks why I want to buy a subway grate. I tell him I love the subway and want one in my apartment as a plant holder. He says that's a new one and gives me the name of the company: Johnson Metal Fabricators in Hamden, Connecticut.

I call and get switched to a salesman, Jim.

He asks, "How many tons of grates you want?"

Shocked, I ask, "Tons?"

"Yeah, the minimum order is one ton, which is twenty grates," he responds.

I mumble, "I need just one."

Jim replies, "Okay, one ton it is. Give me your contact info, and you can pick them up in three weeks."

I clarify, "I just need one, as in one grate."

Jim snickers, "Nobody's gonna sell you one grate. What the hell are you going to do with just one grate?"

I decide to come clean and explain that I want to recreate the famous subway scene with Marilyn Monroe.

He stops me there. "I loved *The Seven Year Itch* and think about that scene a lot. I can't sell you a single grate, but I can give you one. Only one catch: Invite me to the show."

"Done" is my response, and I pick up the grate the next day.

Next, I need to concoct something that mimics the wind blowing up through my subway grate. At this point, I'm several days into no-sleep land and can see the end (of me) is near. I give Keith, the most talented carpenter I have ever known, a call and explain my predicament.

He sighs wistfully, "I loved that scene. Every time I walk by a subway grate, I hope a babe with a flowy dress will walk over it just as the subway passes by." He adds, "But for the record, that babe's my Lovely Wife." He promises he will handle everything, including delivering it to the event, with just one just one catch: "I want two tickets to the event, and a room for the night, for my Lovely Wife and me."

"Done and done," I agree.

Time is ticking away with a month remaining until the big event. I'm flat out, no sleep, and multiprocessing the many things left to complete. I'm beyond salvage, irrational, and, well, crazy. Those around me know that I'm off the rails, yet somehow I convince them that the show must go on, at least I think I do. At 4:00 a.m., my head fills with numbers, more and more numbers: pi out to ten places, Avogadro's number (6.023×10^{23}), Euler's number (e) out to fifteen places, and on and on.

Finally, the number 90°N. Hmm. It's the first number containing a letter. I realize it is a polar coordinate, and not just any polar coordinate, but one that pinpoints the North Pole. That is the sign I have been waiting for: the final showdown with Voldemort will be at the North Pole. Then I pass out.

CHAPTER 3

"I WANT MRCLEAN HOSPITAL. THAT'S WHERE JAMES TAYLOR WENT"

DAY 1, TUESDAY, JULY 31

I am jolted awake by Lovely Wife pushing me through a warren of hallways, in a wheelchair, finally ending up in my psychiatrist's office at "MorAss General Hospital." I hear muffled voices and realize my business partner is also present. I sort of remember that I was scheduled to see my psychiatrist today. However, I was concerned there might be a conflict among the group. Over the previous few months, my hypomania, a less severe form of mania, had progressively worsened as the dosage of my medication was being increased. There seemed to be a positive correlation.

This led me to surmise that the medication was making my condition worse, not better. I had convinced my partner that there might be some merit to my hypothesis, and he had agreed to attend the meeting. I might have also casually mentioned something about trying to get my doctor's license revoked, or at least suspended, which understandably alarmed both Lovely Wife and business partner. Lovely Wife vehemently disagrees with my assessment, reminding me that my doctor is one of the top psychiatrists in the country, if not the top. According to her, my doctor believed that the increasing dosage wasn't able to keep up with my rapidly escalating mania, not an unreasonable counterhypothesis.

With everything spiraling out of control, and to avert a nasty showdown, I do the natural thing: I fake a spastic seizure. With my arms flailing, head rocking back and forth, I put on quite a show. At the end of my act, to signal Lovely Wife that everything was okay, I flashed her the Junior Birdman gesture. For those unfamiliar with it, the gesture involves creating an "okay" sign with each hand, then placing your hands over your eyes, upside down with palms facing your face. I did this a lot when I was young and, then again, not so young. As I start to lose consciousness once again, I can hear the lyrics to the Birdman song:

Up in the air, Junior Birdman
Flying so high off the ground,
Is it a bird, plane, or Superman?
No! It's Junior Birdman upside down.

"Up in the Air, Junior Birdman,"
Junior Birdmen of America Club, 1934

The next thing I remember is being in MorAss General's emergency psych ward, strapped onto a gurney. Two nurses are discussing what to do with me. I overhear one suggest that I get an MRI to see if there is something structurally wrong with my brain.

I interrupt, "No fucking way I'm getting an MRI. I'm claustrophobic, and my head will explode."

They confer again and agree—no MRI. The nurse assigned as my handler states that fortunately there is one bed open in the ward, and they can admit me.

Again, I object. "No, I want MrClean Hospital. That's where James Taylor went, and I really like his songs." They inform me that I have had a serious psychotic break, and it is no laughing matter.

World-famous MrClean was founded in 1811 and nonwokily named "Asylum for the Insane." No sugarcoating it—in those days they called it the way it was.

The nurses conference again, return, and say, "Okay, the last bed here just got taken. You can be transported to MrClean tomorrow. Tonight, you go into the safe room." Hmm, the safe room—sure it is.

Before being led to the safe room, the nurses remove anything that can be used to do myself in—you aren't allowed to use the "S" word, which rhymes with "collide." They confiscate the usual suspects, and then some: my belt, shoelaces and shoes, pants (apparently you can hang yourself with them), glasses (you might use a lens to cut yourself), shirt (the sleeves could be used as a noose), wallet, watch, phone, and keys. They are all placed in a large Ziploc plastic bag, like the ones you see on police shows when someone gets thrown in jail. Come to think of it, I am being incarcerated, and I'm sure there's a camera filming.

Even the strings on my gown are removed—wait, they snatch the gown as well. I am basically naked, except for my undies. Though, I suppose if I want to, I could stuff my Uniqlo underwear down my throat—a quick but smelly and unhappy ending.

The room itself contains no sharp edges, with smooth, soundproof walls and a one-way mirror similar to those seen in police interrogation rooms on TV cop shows. After they close the doorknob-less door, I settle onto the mattress and see the one thing that might drive me to the brink: the president who shall not be named, on Fox News.

I hadn't noticed at first, but the TV set is turned on outside my room and is visible through a window in the top corner of the room, opposite the bed. I find myself face-to-face with a malevolence that is second only to Voldemort, maybe tied. A wannabe dictator and narcissist of the highest order. He should be in this room, not me.

I start to sweat as the room suddenly gets smaller and smaller; after all, I am clinically claustrophobic. I'm locked in, and I can't turn off the damn TV. There's no remote—I guess they think I might swallow the batteries. I must get that TV off, and NOW. I recall the nurses mentioning that if I need help, I should push the button—the red one behind the bed, mounted flush to the wall. I press the button, a red light starts blinking outside the room, and I wave frantically at a nurse.

She rushes in and asks in a concerned voice, "What's wrong?"

I tell her, only half-jokingly, "You forgot to remove the one thing that might drive me to kill myself—having to look at HIS face all night long."

Bad choice of words. The joke was on me as she seems to enter "suicidal ideation" into my record. Thankfully, she does turn off the TV. Note to self: Psych wards are no place for humor. Within a couple of minutes, a nurse gives me a handful of pills. She watches as I swallow them one at a time, and I'm out.

CHAPTER 4

"YOU PAY FOR IT ONE WAY OR ANOTHER"

DAY 2: WEDNESDAY, AUGUST 1

I'm jostled awake as the ambulance rounds a turn. Once again, I find myself strapped into a gurney, this time held down in a straitjacket-like restraint. Rather than self-harm, they may be more worried about harm to the EMT riding next to me. If I were feeling generous, I might say the straitjacket is to prevent me from falling out on the turns, but I'm not feeling generous. As I've mentioned before, I am morbidly claustrophobic, and being trapped in a straitjacket ranks among my worst fears, perhaps tied with being waterboarded. Straitjackets often feature in my nightmares.

Toward the end of the twenty-minute drive, the EMT starts up a conversation.

"First time?" he asks.

"First time for what?" I respond.

"First time going to 'Summer Camp'?"

"Summer Camp?" I ask, perplexed.

He laughs. "That's what we euphemistically call the nuthouse."

"Yeah, first time."

I suddenly realize this is not your average EMT. Anyone who uses "euphemistically," a fifteen-letter word, must have an interesting backstory. It turns out he's an aspiring author who has written his first, as-yet unpublished novel. It's about a time-traveling doctor who uses future medical breakthroughs to save past lives.

Sounds like a medical twist on the *Back to the Future* plot. With an "almost there," he gives me some advice.

"At the admitting window, answer yes to the question, 'Are you voluntarily being admitted?' It will make it easier for you as you navigate the various bureaucratic and legal hassles ahead." I decide to take his advice.

I decide to ask him one last question before we arrive. "Exactly what should I expect on the inside?"

He responds, "Well, you are one of the lucky ones. MrClean is the best psychiatric hospital in the country. They are always booked, and you basically have to be really rich, know someone, or get extremely lucky."

I guess I know someone, or at least Lovely Wife does—she always does. "In any event, the state hospitals are really bad; some even have rapists and murderers as patients."

On that happy note, we arrive at MrClean Hospital. They transfer me into a wheelchair and guide me through a wide, heavy metal door into the admitting area. The door closes behind me with an ominous *clunk*. They unstrap me and help me to my feet, and I notice I'm still in my Uniqlos. I'm led to a counter where a bored-looking clerk asks me if I'm a voluntary or involuntary admission. When I answer, "voluntary," she hands me a stack of papers and tells me to sign on the proverbial dotted lines—about fifty of them. I have no idea exactly what I'm signing, but it looks like MrClean can do pretty much whatever they want to me, whenever they want.

The EMT, who I notice was waiting, hands my bag of belongings to a waiting nurse who assures me it will be kept "in a safe place." They hand me a short-sleeve, buttonless PJ top and pants with an elastic waist band to change into.

"Send him to Ward B South, room 21B," the admitting nurse instructs.

Still in the wheelchair, I'm taken in the elevator to the second floor, then through two more sets of doors, each shutting behind with the same secure *clunk*. The corridor between them is monitored by two security cameras, one at each end. Once again, I'm reminded of a prison scene. Finally, I enter Ward B South, where a smiling nurse greets us.

She turns to the other nurse: "I'll take it from here."

The nurse wheels me down a hallway, where I glimpse a couple of the other inmates. One is sitting with a blank look on her face. Wait a minute, HER face. I'm thinking THEY, the ones running the asylum, are the crazy ones. I can't be the only manic one here, and isn't hypersexuality one of the most widely acknowledged symptoms? The other inmate is standing, with a blank look on his face—wait a minute, he looks to be just seventeen years old. How many pedophiles might there be in Ward B South? I shake my head in disbelief.

I'm taken to room 21B, where the nurse gestures toward the bed on the right. On the left is my new roommate. The nurse doesn't introduce us, and my roommate doesn't even acknowledge my presence. In this new world, I figure it makes sense. Is he psycho? Does he think I am psycho? We are probably both psychos, hence, the nickname, Psycho Ward. I wonder, Does professional courtesy hold?

None of this makes any sense. So, who do you call? *Seinfeld.* I think back to one of my favorite episodes, or at least what I can remember of it through the fog of heavy-duty drugs. It's the one where George Costanza works for George Steinbrenner of Yankees fame. Every decision Costanza makes—personnel, financial, even down to which towel to use in the locker room—turns out to be exactly wrong. His unconventional solution is do the exact opposite of his first instinct. Steinbrenner is so happy with this reinvented Costanza that he becomes Steinbrenner's new "superstar" for consistently "knocking it out of the park." I'm gonna go with it.

As I survey the room, I see no curtains, dressers, or anything with sharp edges, just a cubbyhole and a pillow, sans case. Instead of making you feel comfortable and putting your mind at ease, they continually remind you of the risk of suicide, and of course one of the biggest triggers for committing the act is to visualize it. "Do you have suicidal ideation?" they will ask. And the likely answer will be, "Well, now I do."

Just then the nurse walks in—something they can always do since the doors neither lock nor even fully close—and informs me that it is time to take my medications. I follow him and join a queue of several other "guests" (I plan to use this term interchangeably with "inmates," "clients," "patients," and "victims") in front of a counter waiting to "take our medicine." I'm third in line. The person in front of me isn't paying attention and doesn't realize it's her turn. I tap her on the shoulder, and all hell breaks loose. She screeches with a chilling, bloodcurdling snarl, "Don't touch me, you motherfucker!" and proceeds to punch me. Several nurses rush over, pull her away, force her pills into her mouth, watch her swallow, and lead her away.

The head nurse runs up to me and sternly says, "Never do that again."

"Do what?" I ask angrily.

"Never touch anyone in this ward. That is rule number one. Some of the patients don't like to be touched, and we don't know who might react that way."

"Oh, nobody told me about that. I tap her on the shoulder, she beats the crap out of me, and it's my fault?"

As she turns to leave, she sneers, "Learn the rules, and it will make things easier for you." As she's walking down the hall, I call out, "There's a simple test to determine if someone doesn't like to be touched: just touch them."

Whoops, big mistake. She rushes to the enclosed nursing station, pulls out my file, and makes an entry. I'm now at the head of the line; the nurse glances at my wrist bracelet, enters a locked room, and emerges with about half a dozen pills in a small paper cup.

I recognize two of them: my blood pressure and statin pills. The others vary in sizes, shapes, and colors. I turn to leave.

"Wait, I need to see you take each one individually and open your mouth afterward, so I can see that you've swallowed them."

I'm tempted to tell her what she can swallow, but I do as she says—more or less. I remember how Jack Nicholson hid his pills in his cheek in *One Flew over the Cuckoo's Nest*, and cheek my last one and leave with a smirk.

As I head back to my room, one of the young female guests walks up to me, gives me a hug, and whispers in my ear, "Don't worry. I'll take care of you and show you how to get out of here."

When the nurse glares at her, she flips him the bird. I sense that we're going to be good friends. She notices that I see the scars on her wrists.

Once in my room, I nod toward my roommate, who, of course, just stares blankly into space. With three hours until dinner, what to do? The only reasonable thing to do is plan my escape. But how? An old idea pops into my head. At the right moment—perhaps in the middle of the night—pull the fire alarm. They'll have to evacuate us, right? Then I'll scram. This trick worked in high school, when the jocks, who never scored high grades but scored with the cheerleaders, would get out of a test by pulling the fire alarm, which required everyone to leave the school until the fire department showed up.

When I arrived, I didn't see any fences surrounding MrClean. In my younger days, I was a nationally ranked marathoner and finished thirteen marathons. I was proud of the fact that if I'd been a female, I would have won the female division of almost every race. Note to self: Ask Lovely Wife to bring me my running sneakers and shorts, ASAP.

A nurse pokes his head in and announces, "You've got a phone call."

Startled, I respond eloquently, "Huh?"

He clarifies, "You've got a phone call at the public phone in the hall around the corner."

Still confused I ask, "Could you please show me? I don't know my way around here yet."

With a "Sure," he leads me down the hall, makes a right turn, and points me to an old-school phone booth, with a small bench seat and no door. The phone is dangling, and when I pick up, it turns out to be Lovely Wife.

She says she is just checking up and will be there sometime after 7:00 p.m. and hangs up before I can mention to bring my running outfit. She clearly sounds relieved that I'm in a safe place, but perhaps not as "safe" as she thinks. As I return the receiver to its cradle, I see a sign in large red lettering above the phone: "This phone is ONLY for incoming calls. HIPAA laws require strict confidentiality." I wonder what tales these phone booth walls would tell if they could. There are a lot of strange birds here, many of them manic and hypersexual, and a phone booth is always a good choice for a forbidden liaison. The "action" may even rival that which occurred in the lavatory on Hugh Hefner's customized DC-9 jet, "Big Bunny."

On the way back to my room, my newfound savior, Kerin, calls over and says, "Dinner is served in fifteen minutes. The doors open at exactly 6:00 p.m. Be there on time, or they'll run out of the turkey, which is the only edible choice." She then whispers, "Let's meet after dinner in the activity room. I'll share my story with you."

I dutifully go to the cafeteria at the suggested time and find a crowd in a somewhat orderly queue. I use the term "queue" since I remember visiting London, where they're particular about their lining up. Given that many Londoners are Oxford and Cambridge graduates, they're aware that "queue" is derived from the Latin word for "tail."

On the other hand, Germans seem to approach lining up as a sport; rugby would be close.

In any event, this line was together enough to go with the English label. Another note to self: Arrive well before 6:00 p.m. next time. Next time? Hmm, I wonder how many "next times" there will be. My stay here is open-ended—some have been here for months—but I can cut it short if I need to with my exit strategy. What worries me is there seems to be something going on that I haven't quite figured out. I hear discussions of a "treatment," and I really don't like the sound of it. The doors swing open, and the line advances toward the entrée counter.

The campers each grab a plastic plate and plastic spoon—no knife or fork, for obvious reasons. The first in line sticks his plate over the glass counter separating the servers from the campers. He points to the turkey and is given a rather miserly helping.

He grunts, "More."

The server sneers, "That's all you get. Next!"

Kerin is on deck and receives her portion, larger than the first guy's. Obviously, assholes get shortchanged. The rest of the line all go with the turkey, gravy, and potatoes. The other two choices are the drastically overcooked fish of indeterminate origin and gray meat, also impossible to classify. The turkey goes fast. However, I am optimistic as the woman directly in front of me gets served turkey.

I step up to the plate and request, with a smile, "Turkey, please."

Her response: "No turkey for you. All gone."

Once again, *Seinfeld* springs to mind. This time the Soup Nazi: "No soup for you!" Henceforth, she will be—wait for it—the Turkey Nazi. I just point to the mashed potatoes and gravy and thank her. One thing I'm certain of is that the food servers rule the ward, whether it be hospital or prison.

Carrying my tray toward the tables, I see Kerin waving me over and pointing to the chair across from her. She cuts her turkey in half with her spoon and gives me half, declaring, "We're a team now." She then adds, "After visiting hour ends at 8:00 p.m., let's meet in the activity room. We can talk then."

Heading back to my room, I wonder who will be visiting me tonight.

Promptly at 7:00 p.m., Lovely Wife heads down the hall—my first visitor. All right, maybe it's more like 7:10 p.m., maybe even 7:15 p.m. She's notoriously late, but always has a good reason. This time, there's a veritable plethora of good reasons: There was bad traffic, the entrance wasn't marked, she had to sign in, her handbag was searched for contraband, she had to navigate a labyrinth of hallways, find the right elevator, and knock on a locked door for several minutes, and finally, there was no official meeting area. I figure the best thing to say is, "Thanks for coming."

Her obligatory first question is, "How's it going?"

I decide to simply respond, "Okay. I actually met someone nice. Her name is Kerin, and she's standing over there. She says she'll help me get out of here."

Lovely Wife waves Kerin over, thanks her, chats her up a bit, then proclaims to me, "You're in good hands. Should I bring you anything tomorrow?"

I request, "My running shoes, running socks, running pants, running hat, and the first and last Harry Potter books."

She responds, "Sure," and heads for the door.

Kerin waves to me and leads me to the activity room. She reveals that she is an aspiring opera singer and is "not too bad." She certainly looks the part, in a young Maria Callas kind of way. Usually when I hear "I am great," the person sucks, but "not too bad" can sometimes mean great. She sees my musing and proceeds to do the "mi, mi, mi, mi" thing that singers do when they warm up. She then belts out "Habanera," the spectacular aria from *Carmen*, made famous by Callas. She sings it in the traditional French, her voice filling the room—no, the entire ward—with perhaps the most beautiful sound I've ever heard.

Here's the second stanza in English:

Love is a gypsy's child,

It has never, ever known a law. Love me not, then I love you.

If I love you, you'd best beware!

She had omitted the fact that she is considered one of the most talented young opera singers of her generation. Not surprisingly, two nurses frantically rush in.

They glare at Kerin and admonish, "You can't sing like that during quiet hours; you can only speak in an indoor voice."

I laugh and say, "You have to admit, it was great."

Then the angry retort, "Both of you are getting written up for rule violation."

We promise to use our indoor voices from now on, and they leave to write their report.

Back to her story. She is a first-year student at Berklee College and the Boston Conservatory. Berklee is considered the world's preeminent college for the study of music—think of it as the Juilliard of voice, based in Boston, with campuses around the world. Their alumni have won a grand total of—wait for it—over three hundred Grammys. Not to mention scores of Oscars, such as Howard Shore's for the music for *Lord of the Rings*; Tonys, including Trey Parker of *Book of Mormon* fame; and Emmys, like Quincy Jones for the music for *Roots*.

Kerin was breaking under the pressure of being the country's next diva. In high school, she had attempted to end her life, hence the scars on her wrists. She has two loving mothers who are tremendously protective of her and didn't want her to leave her native Ohio. She had told them that she "was going to go for it and see where it leads." Well, it led to MrClean, renowned for its rich history of music graduates.

She proceeds to give me a primer on the daily routine. There are three meals a day: breakfast from 7:00 a.m. to 8:00 a.m., lunch from noon to

1:00 p.m., then dinner from 6:00 p.m. to 7:00 p.m. The cafeteria remains open until 8:00 p.m. Breakfast consists of cereal and scrambled eggs, lunch is always sandwiches (turkey being the best choice), and dinner, except for the turkey, crap.

If you are vegan, you'll go even crazier than you were before. Drinks are provided all day. There is powdered hot chocolate, skim milk, and half and half. The good news is that coffee is served all day; the bad news? Only decaf after 4:00 p.m. Caffeine, in my opinion, is one of the most powerful drugs for mental health. It helps with focus, lifts the spirits, keeps you awake—a good thing when driving—and helps you deal with stress.

So, I will get my caffeine, and it will help me remain sane. Hopefully, it will also counteract the drugs they give me to render me complacent and pliable. Getting around the caffeine ban should be easy. I will take two cups of coffee back to my room before the 4:00 p.m. deadline. Then, any time after the deadline, I'll return to the cafeteria and use the microwave to heat it to the optimal 145 degrees Fahrenheit temperature, about sixty-six seconds. However, to offset the bitterness of stale coffee, I'll add hot chocolate mix and concoct a delicious mocha.

At 7:55 p.m., they issue the "Get to your rooms—it's bedtime" command. So, I dutifully return to room 21B, where my roommate is already asleep. Fortunately, I can go straight to sleep after consuming a considerable amount of caffeine. Interestingly, it's like giving Adderall to someone who is hyperactive: It calms them down. Mania is a first cousin to ADHD. I can't wait to start my caffeine therapy tomorrow.

I lie in bed thinking not about how I got here, but rather how to get out. If I simply play by the rules, I could probably get out in a week. Yet, that might just be wishful thinking, given that most prisoners, on average, are in for at least a month, some for over a year. However, I am not average. My grandson is due to be born in the next couple of days, and my only chance to be there depends on my escape, for which I'm formulating a most excellent plan. Hence, I am left with two choices: Play nice and be stuck here for a while and miss my grandson's birth, or take the risky path of an early escape, with serious potential consequences. This is the epitome of a dilemma; I will have to "pay for it one way or another." Suddenly, that phrase sparks a memory, indelibly etched into my brain: "You pay for it one way or another."

It was the mid-1970s. I had just moved to New York City to begin my investment career at one of the top financial institutions in the world. I was among the first "quants" they'd hired. A quant is someone who uses computer algorithms to profit from irrational investors who price stocks on emotion rather than on data. On the other hand, I irrationally decided to spend over half my income on an amazing apartment on the Upper East Side, which was THE place to live in those days. I figured I had everything going for me: not bad looking, a six-pack, good hair, a great job, a sense of humor, a killer apartment, and no excessive body odor or earwax. Bottom line: In those days, I would have been described as a "chick slayer." Don't judge me for that—those times were different. It was the tail end of the *Mad Men* era.

I got my reality check my first week in the city. I went out solo to the hot bar on the Upper East Side—J.G. Melon. I arrived at about 10:00 p.m. and ordered a beer. I was checking out the crowd when a nice-looking, friendly guy started chatting me up.

"I haven't seen you here before. Are you new to the neighborhood? How's it going? You live in the city?"

At this point, I was getting a little weirded out.

This guy was not someone with whom I wished to intercourse—the second definition, meaning to converse. Suddenly, I felt a hand down my pants. I turned around to see if it was one of the hotties at the bar—paydirt. Much to my shock, disbelief, and chagrin, it was the guy who had approached me. Apparently, he was interested in the first definition of intercourse. I made a quick exit and headed home, dejected.

Reflecting on this now triggers a deeply repressed memory from even earlier, 1968. These flashbacks must be the result of my medications. I was fifteen, and more than a little bit socially awkward. Insecure, with Coke bottle glasses, not a good look. For the ophthalmologists out there, my vision was 14 diopters—that's 20/2000 vision.

To put that into perspective, what I could see at a distance of twenty feet, a normal eye could see at two thousand feet. How bad was that?

Legally blind is 20/200, so ten times worse than legally blind. Contact lenses were not an option, as they weren't available. I wasn't just kissless—I hadn't even held hands with someone other than a relative, and come to think of it, maybe not even that.

December rolled around, and the big social scene was going ice skating at the Willow Grove Ice Skating Rink. I went there occasionally with my likewise vision-impaired, nerdy friends. We'd stand at one end of the rink while the popular crowd congregated at the other end. The popular group consisted mostly of jocks and the pretty, "fast" girls, mostly cheerleaders with nicknames like "Pompom" and "Twirl." The biggest difference between their group and ours was the presence of girls. We had none on our side, not even the nerdy girls; they would have rather stayed home than be seen with us. Nevertheless, being clever, I sought to change that predicament. I needed a date, ideally someone who could also skate.

The only strategy that I thought might help in this situation was John Nash's theory on how to pick up a beautiful girl at a bar, even if you are a nerd. Nash was a brilliant mathematician who specialized in a branch of economics called game theory. He proposed to his socially awkward friends at Princeton that the only way any of them of them stood a chance of attracting the prettiest girl in a bar was for everyone in the nerd group to ignore her and focus their attention on the other girls.

Eventually, the most desirable girl, now ignored, would start wondering why the nerds were overlooking her and might feel compelled to join the conversation. She might begin to think, Maybe there's more to these guys than meets the eye, and pick one to conquer.

Even though the odds of any individual from the nerdy group winning the prize were just 1/n—with n being the number of nerds—it was significantly better than zero. For the mathematically challenged, if there are four nerds, any one of them would have a one-in-four chance of success. Of course, this was all theoretical. Ironically, Nash also did a stint at MrClean.

However, that strategy wouldn't work for me since I was only fifteen and six years away from being allowed into a bar. But at least Nash gave me hope that nerds could score. So, I came up with the "law of comparative advantage for getting a hot date." My comparative advantage was that I was a high school sophomore. In my school district, high school included grades 10 through 12, so being a sophomore may have been at the bottom of the pecking order there, but I was still in the big leagues. On the other hand, junior high covered grades 7 through 9, with a seventh grader being at the bottom of the minor leagues.

My theory suggested that a seventh grader would jump at the chance to go out with a high school guy. If I dipped down three grades, I should have my pick. Fortunately, one of the seventh graders lived nearby, the sister of a classmate. Even though the older sister would never consider dating me, she thought I was smart and harmless. I figured that Diane would give me a positive recommendation, if asked.

This seventh grader, Sweet Sue, was a perfect ten. She would wear miniskirts so short they could be called microskirts, and she had the best legs that nature ever created. In my school district, Cheltenham Township, the administration tried to control the ever-shorter skirts the girls were wearing. They even passed a rule stating that a skirt could not be more than eight inches above the knee. However, Sweet Sue found a way around it. After the homeroom teacher measured the skirts of all the miniskirted girls, Sweet Sue would head to the girls' restroom before her first class and roll her skirt at the waist a couple of turns.

Magically, her skirt was a good ten inches above her knees: genius. She was not just hot, but twenty-seven million degrees hot, the temperature in the middle of the sun. The rest of the package was just as good, and she was smart. Now my first hurdle was that I would never directly ask a girl on a date, given my extreme fear of rejection. Luckily, the girl next door happened to also be in seventh grade and knew Sweet Sue.

I asked Sandy if she knew whether Sue liked to ice-skate.

"Loves it."

I queried, "Could you ask her if she would meet me at Willow Grove Ice Skating Rink Friday night?"

"Sure."

I received a yes. First problem solved.

The second problem was that the Willow Grove Ice Skating Rink was five miles away, and I couldn't drive yet. My parents would have gladly driven me, but I didn't want them clued in, so I told them I was going to the racetrack with my best friend Larry, who was a year older and had a driver's license. We went to Brandywine Racetrack in Delaware quite a bit, since they didn't check your ID. I loved to beat the odds and hoped for a long shot this Friday night. Sweet Sue's parents agreed to drop her off and pick her up.

The solution to the second problem was to hitchhike. In those days it was very common; I did it all the time, and even my parents knew. Sweet Sue and I were to meet at 7:00 p.m. Since I didn't know exactly how long it would take me, I allowed an hour—being late was not an option. I got there with no problem, with just one ride, arriving thirty minutes early. That turned out to be less than optimal, since it gave me enough time to have a panic attack.

Thankfully, when she arrived, I saw that she was wearing one of her trademark miniskirts. Not the micro version but the more conservative, regulation mini, about eight inches above her knee. In my Spanish class, I learned the appropriate expression to describe the vision before me, "muy caliente," and may have even mumbled it. Fortunately, she took French.

We nervously chatted for a while before heading to the skate rental desk. We got our skates, I gladly paid, then we put them on and headed to the rink. The popular group was at the three o'clock part of the rink, and as usual, the nerds were across the rink at nine o'clock. Because I didn't want to reveal I was one of the nerds, we went directly onto the ice. After a couple of circuits around the rink, I decided to take the plunge. I held out my hand and—wait for it—she took it. That moment is indelibly etched into my mind. You never forget your first handhold.

We passed the nerds first; they were stunned. Better yet, as we passed the popular group, the girls immediately cast their eyes on their new competition. I saw looks of shock on their faces: Who the hell was this stunning intruder in their territory? The boys, naturally, were drooling. Even better, next to her, and holding her hand was me, the recovering nerd.

Best night of my life, and I learned another valuable lesson. Along with the Nash method of meeting pretty girls, with my "dip three grades down" gambit, I found another winning strategy: Be seen with the hottest girl, and all the other hot girls will want you. They'll figure that there must be more to the book than the cover. Having said that, I guess that was actually a Nash variation. The rest of the night went by quickly. I was in a trance—no, make that an alternate universe.

I was plummeted back to earth when Sweet Sue said, "I have to go. My parents are outside."

As she turned away, she said, "I had a really nice time."

I had to hustle home. It was getting late. I'd told my parents I'd be back from the track at about 10:00 p.m. I headed for Willow Grove Avenue and stuck out my thumb. The first car passing by jammed on its brakes and pulled over.

A man in his thirties smiled and asked, "Where are you going?"

I replied, "Lynwood Gardens Apartments, Washington Lane and Ashbourne Avenue."

He said, "That's on my way. Hop in."

After about three miles, he turned off Washington Lane and took a detour into Curtis Arboretum, a park that was usually deserted at night. It had once been the estate of the founder of Curtis Publishing, with gardens designed by Frederick Law Olmsted, of Central Park fame, that later became the arboretum. This definitely was not right. While the car was still moving, I felt a hand on my thigh, then on my privates. He began to rub and squeeze aggressively. I didn't panic but was acutely aware of the danger. I glanced to my right and saw that the door was unlocked. The choice between "fight or flight" was easy; he was twice my size. FLIGHT.

I opened the door while the car was moving at about twenty miles per hour and jumped. I rolled a few times, stood up, and ran like hell.

As he was getting out of his car, he yelled, "Fuck you, you bastard!"

Even back then I was a very good runner, so I turned, gave him the finger, and managed to make it home on time. My parents didn't ask any questions or notice anything wrong. I haven't told this story until now.

Now, back to New York, circa the 1970s. After the second sexual assault of my life at J.G. Melon, I avoided going out for quite a while. It wasn't that I was afraid—I could have beaten the shit out of the guy who molested me—but I was just dejected. A few months passed, and one night after working late, I left the office around 9:00 p.m. and crossed the plaza outside my building—it actually was THE Plaza, as in the famous Plaza Hotel, on Fifty-Ninth Street and Fifth Avenue. Out of the corner of my eye, I noticed someone approaching me at a 45-degree angle, moving at a fast pace, obviously trying to intercept me.

I took a quick glance over my shoulder and liked what I saw. I still remember the details: very attractive, dark auburn hair parted to the side, dark pink lipstick, red nail polish, well-dressed in a red knee-length tailored dress showing just an inch or two of ample cleavage, in her mid-twenties with a beautiful, angelic smile. I slowed down, and she caught up with me. I detected the subtle aroma of perfume, perhaps Chanel. I knew Chanel, since as a stock analyst I covered the cosmetics companies.

She inquired in an alluring voice, "Do you want to party?"

Instantly, I thought, *Now this is what I'm talking about*, and replied, "That sounds good."

She then proceeded to inform me how much the different entrees being served at the party would cost. "Hand job, twenty-five dollars; tit fuck, thirty-five dollars; vaginal sex, fifty dollars; anal, seventy-five dollars; and the special of the day, an anything-goes threesome for one hundred and fifty bucks."

I was shocked as well as not certain what some of the entrees actually were. It was not what I was hoping for, and I blurted out, "I don't pay for sex."

She immediately responded, with a big grin, "Sweetie, you pay for it one way or another."

Back to the question, whether to just do my time in the ward or flee. I opt for the quick escape option and vow to come up with a more concrete plan tomorrow. I fall asleep at 10:00 p.m., only to be awoken at 10:15 by the glare of a flashlight hitting my eyes. It's the nurse opening the door to check in on me.

I bolt upright and ask, "What the hell are you doing?"

He says he just wants to make sure I'm okay. I mumble something and then go back to sleep. Then at 10:30, the same thing happens, although this time I say nothing. 10:45, same. 11:00, same

The pattern now becomes clear: They check in every fifteen minutes. I'm on SUICIDE watch—just like they depict in the cop shows.

At 11:16, the door opens, and I say, "You're a minute late. By the way, do you have a suggestion box?"

He whispers, "Yeah, over by the main desk in the middle of the ward." I stumble out of bed, go to the desk, and find a box with a slot, some paper, and, of course, a crayon labeled "edible."

I write out my complaint: "I keep getting woken up every fifteen minutes or so. Perhaps it might make sense to let me sleep. To the best of my knowledge, I have not been diagnosed as someone who might inflict harm upon himself."

CHAPTER 5

"MENTAL ILLNESS DOES NOT TAKE WEEKENDS OFF"

DAY 3: THURSDAY, AUGUST 2

On and on it goes. I feel a bit like Sisyphus, the Greek king doomed to repeatedly roll the same boulder up a hill, for eternity. Every fifteen minutes, my folded complaints get shorter: "Please stop," then "Stop." Finally, "STOP," and in total frustration, I take a bite out of the crayon and toss it into the box.

At 6:30 a.m., I hear on the intercom, "Breakfast will begin at 7:00 a.m. Please get ready."

I decide to make one last trip to the suggestion box and write, "You suck." I head back to my room, smiling, head held high, and, according to their report, naked.

Into the hallway I go. I grab a towel from a table and head to the bathroom to shower, shave, and do my business.

A female nurse intercepts me and frantically says, "You can't go into the bathroom alone. You must have a male nurse observing."

I glance toward the bathroom door and see the male nurse, Jason, standing there, supervising the bathroom traffic.

I'm second in line. Surprisingly, things go quickly as the person in front of me leaves after just a few minutes. Jason waves me to follow him in and offers to walk me through the bathroom protocol. He wants to know my routine.

After a little thought, I present him with my plan. First, hit the toilet, then wash my hands, brush my teeth, shower, towel off, shave, wash face, towel off again, and finish with a comb through my hair. Why that order, you ask? Doing your business is gross, so you need to wash your hands immediately. Brushing your teeth can mess up your hands, face, and chin, so the shower will clean both up. Shaving is easier with a warm, softened beard, so that goes last. Finally, a comb through the hair to look good, or at least better.

Now for the reality of this place. I don't have my toothbrush—I thought, like in a hotel, one would be supplied. I'll ask Lovely Wife to bring me one when she visits tonight. The toilet stall lacks a door, and the toilet paper is just a roll on the floor—for safety reasons, I presume. The toilet doesn't have a handle; it is an automatic one that flushes as I stand up to leave. I don't see the shower, so I ask Jason where it is.

"Over there by the wall."

There is no curtain, no handles to control the water, and the shower-head hangs from the ceiling about eight feet above the floor, perhaps to prevent you from hanging yourself with a towel? The shower is triggered by a motion sensor. I don't see the soap, but I do see Jason walking over with one of those foaming soap dispensers. He informs me that it is an all-purpose soap, suitable for both body and hair, and he'll dispense as much as I need into my hands, but just once. I request a generous portion, "Keep it coming," and proceed with my usual shower routine: washing my hair and then working my way down. Why do I use this technique so religiously?

Well, my efficiency engineer father always said that the best way to wash a car was from the top down, to prevent the dirt from above soiling the cleaned sections below, with the wheels last. He'd add, "Showering is the same."

Maxi was right. I finish with my "wheels," my feet. I towel off, wrap the towel around me, and inquire about shaving.

Jason informs me, "You can't shave today. We have to make sure it's safe before we give you a razor."

I retort, "But it's called a safety razor."

I can guess at the answer to the next one. I ask, "How about a comb for my hair?"

He laughs, "That's a no."

On my way back to my room, I grab a fresh pair of brown PJs from a huge stack in the corner. I optimistically choose medium. A tight fit, but my ego requires it.

I sit alone in a corner for breakfast; it is uneventful. However, I do notice the aroma of the food cooking, especially the strong smell of bacon sizzling on the stovetop, which provides a nice contrast to the antiseptic scent of chlorine that fills the rest of the ward. I head back to my room to flesh out my escape plan. I'm intercepted by a nurse who tells me that it's time for me to take my medicine. I stroll up to the window, thankfully without incident, and notice a significantly fuller cup of pills than yesterday and wonder what they are. I'm aware that medicines can be either fat soluble or water soluble. Fat-soluble medicines stay in the body longer, and the blood concentration can rise precipitously if the dose is too high. On the other hand, if you miss one, it is not that big a deal.

Conversely, water-soluble medications get washed out of the body quickly through your urine, making dosing trickier. It's generally better to administer these pills several times a day rather than in one dose to avoid the yo-yo effect, where the blood concentration is too high right after you take them and too low just before you take the next dose.

So, to clarify, I ask the nurse which pills are water soluble and which are fat soluble.

She shakes her head and says, "I have no idea."

"Perhaps you can call one of the doctors?"

She retorts, "First you will have to see the pharmacist, who will write up a request to the doctor. However, she won't see it until Monday."

Puzzled, I ask, "Why Monday?"

She replies condescendingly, "The weekend is coming up. The doctors don't work weekends."

I respond sharply, "Mental illness does not take weekends off."

I get written up, told to take the pills, and then directed to another nursing station down the hall, where they will take my vitals. I tell myself that I will have to use that catchy phrase again.

As it turns out, "vitals" include sucking my blood out with a needle.

I detest needles. I inform the nurse that I sometimes pass out when I have blood drawn.

She smiles and whispers soothingly, "Don't worry. It will be okay."

Don't worry. Yeah, sure. I decide to educate her on why needles are the instrument of the devil to me.

"When I was seven," I begin, "I was playing on a playground near our apartment."

In the 1950s, playgrounds didn't have the soft, cushy ground covering we have today. Instead, they were covered with macadam, also known as blacktop, the stuff they use to pave roads today. It was hard, smelly, build to last twenty-five years, and might reach 140 degrees Fahrenheit in the sun. It was a form of childhood Darwinism—"only the toughest survived."

I climbed up the stairs of a towering, seven-foot-high slide. Just as I reached the top, the neighborhood bully decided that I was obstructing his fun and pushed me off. The next thing I knew, I was in the hospital.

People were rushing around. I heard whispering: "He's lost a lot of blood—that's what happens with head wounds."

They propped me up, and the doctor grabbed a gigantic hypodermic needle from a jar filled with alcohol. In those days, needles were reused and stored that way to keep them sterile.

The needle was long and thick; they didn't have the thin pediatric ones they use today. The doctor mumbled something about giving me a shot to numb the pain when he "sews me up." He steadied my head with his left hand and plunged the needle in with his right.

"Shit!" he exclaimed. It was the first time I'd ever heard a curse word, although I didn't know what one was at the time.

He called for the nurse to fetch a hemostat, a plier-like instrument, and proceeded to yank the snapped-off needle from my head. I broke into a cold sweat and threw up on the doctor.

Flash-forward to the present. The color drains out of the nurse's face. She suggests that it would be best for me to return in the afternoon. As I'm leaving, I see her scribbling some notes.

I head back to my room to find my roommate has moved out without saying a word, true to character. The nurse informs me that I'll get a new one tomorrow. I appreciate the quiet and use the next few hours before lunch to solve the "doctors don't work weekends" problem. It doesn't take long. Automobile plants had come up with a solution long ago.

When cars are in high demand, they operate 24/7. They employ "shift work." I use a variant of their plan to sketch out mine.

In hospitals, they seem to employ linear thinking. Most doctors, at least those here, work Monday through Friday, taking weekends off. The problem is, as I pointed out earlier, mental illness does not take weekends off, it doesn't take nights off, and it doesn't take lunch hours off; it is 24/7/365/until you die. I can't solve all the lunacy here, but I can solve the weekend issue.

Let's suppose we have seven doctors. Since I don't have anything to draw with, I start visualizing the solution; I'll physically sketch it out later. It's faster this way, anyway. I envision a circle with seven equally spaced points around its perimeter. Each point is labeled with a day of the week, going clockwise: Monday, Tuesday, Wednesday, Thursday, Friday, Saturday, Sunday—M, Tu, W, Th, F, Sa, Su for short.

I then connect the Monday through Friday points; it is an arc on the circle. Then it gets interesting. The next two arcs are Tuesday thru Saturday and Wednesday thru Sunday, and so on. With this scheme, each doctor gets two consecutive days off, and weekends are fully staffed.

The biggest hurdle for adoption: They didn't think about it, and it's not how it is being done. On the way to my room, I spot a small box of crayons and quickly draw out my idea. I submit my simple yet elegant solution to one of the nurses just before lunch. I see her write a short note and file it under, "He is exhibiting delusions of grandeur and thinks he knows better," I'm sure.

Kerin invites me to lunch. Hopefully, she will become my regular meal date. We observe how the nurses spend much more time in their central hub than on the ward tending to us, which you would think is their primary job. This hub, which I've nicknamed Grand Central Station, sits at the intersection of three hallways. With glass walls, we can see everything they are doing and vice versa—Latin for "the other way around." Our rooms and bathrooms are located down these hallways.

Two of the hallways have five guest rooms each—four doubles and one single. The third hallway is a somewhat of a mystery, featuring just four single rooms. The occupants never leave that hallway. Nobody seems to know exactly what happens there, but no one wants to end up there. Is it solitary confinement, or even death row? Maybe both. Adding it all up, there are a total of twenty-two guests on the ward. It is rare for a room to remain vacant for more than a few hours, a day at most. There is always a wait-list to get in: When one customer leaves, another takes their place, like a queue at a popular restaurant. Occasionally, I hear a nurse on the phone say, "Sorry, we are fully committed," or words to that effect.

The nurses are almost always at their desks, which face the glass walls, engrossed in their computers. It's clear they're documenting the behavior and activities of the guests, perhaps even minute by minute. I notice a pattern: Following nearly every interaction with me, they hurry back to their desk, typing furiously. I assume that can't be a good thing.

As a student of cognitive dissonance, or its sibling, confirmation bias, if you have a prior belief—say, for example, *This patient really needs our help. He continues to exhibit erratic behavior, and we must watch him very carefully because he is a clear and present danger not only to himself, but also society at large. Most importantly, he looks litigious, so we must document everything to cover our asses*—cognitive dissonance will prevent you from considering any evidence that contradicts this belief. Confirmation bias is similar, but rather than excluding evidence, in this case an individual seeks out only evidence that supports their preexisting belief.

The smarter you are, the harder you fall for it, making it virtually impossible to alter your view. Now, to be fair, there is plenty of evidence that I do need serious help—after all, I am convinced that I am the leader of the existential fight between good and evil. However, I often make the nurses laugh and smile with my witty banter. I don't throw either my food during meals or a punch when lining up for my meds, and I haven't uttered a single curse word, at least out loud, I'm pretty sure.

Lunch ends, and Kerin, now appraised of my escape plan, suggests that she might have an item in her room that could trigger the fire alarm, providing the necessary distraction for my escape. She will leave it on the shelf in her room, to the left, just inside the door. On my way to my temporarily single room, I spot a fire alarm near the emergency exit and examine it carefully.

There is no obvious way to set it off, no handle to pull or button to push—that would be too easy. I notice a keyhole, but they wouldn't design a fire alarm to operate only with a key, would they? They might. I deduce that smoke or CO_2 probably sets it off.

I presume Kerin's "something" is something that emits CO_2. I go down the hall to her room; she's not there. I go in and grab the container she described, which contains—wait for it—moisturizing cream. It gets worse: I don't notice that Kerin's roommate is in the room.

She starts screaming, "Man in the room! Man in the room!"

At this point, two sizable male nurses burst in, grab me by the arms, and forcefully escort me back to my room. They shut the door, and the larger nurse stands guard outside. I am certain the other nurse is heading back to his computer to write this one up, and maybe summon one of the doctors. I know I'm in BIG trouble.

About fifteen minutes later, the two male nurses escort me to the ominous secret hallway, the land of no return, where the worst of the worst are warehoused, and into the one empty room.

The door shuts behind me, just as one of the nurses says, "I'll be back in a couple of minutes with something to help your condition."

I don't think I have a condition, just caught in the act, but I figure I don't have much of a case for not taking my medicine.

I mentally go through a list of things that I've done that may have been considered a little outside the norm. Touching the girl in line for her pills and precipitating a fight, writing forty-three complaints about the glaring lights in my face on my first night, bitching about doctors taking the weekend off and diagramming my eloquent solution, and bursting into a girl's room to snatch moisturizing cream. I wasn't exactly wrong about all of these, except for the moisturizing cream thing. Perhaps apologizing and claiming my skin was getting dry could help. However, bottom line, I can see how an outside observer might find my behavior a bit aberrant—no, make that downright crazy.

Five minutes pass, and the nurse returns to give me the "help"—three enormous pills that are hard to swallow, one at a time. He says he will return in about an hour. It doesn't take long before I feel my free will slowly draining away. I am here, but not present. When he returns, I am completely complacent, probably for the first time in my life. I can hear, but not speak. The antidote, my mocha, is out of reach for now.

The nurse begins, "Do you know why you are here?"

Now able to speak, albeit very slowly, I mumble, "Because I asked for a single room?"

The nurse says, "Look, let me give it to you straight. I actually like you, especially that you don't really give a shit about the rules. I also think some of the rules are stupid. However, you've ticked off the hierarchy who manage this place, particularly your doctor. She runs this place." He continues, "She's in charge of your case, and here's the deal: She can pretty much treat you however she wants. Your psychiatrist has no jurisdiction here."

For some reason, I have a flashback to Nurse Ratched, the villainous "caregiver" from *One Flew over the Cuckoo's Nest*, and blurt out, "Dr. Ratched?"

"How bad is that?" I ask cautiously.

He continues ominously, "Dr. Ratched, as you call her, can order ECT for you." ECT stands for electroconvulsive therapy, renamed from the more accurate electroconvulsive shock therapy.

Shocked myself, I utter, "First, I didn't know they still performed that, especially after *Cuckoo's Nest*. I've heard rumors about it, but isn't it just for treatment-resistant depression?"

He responds somberly, "No, it's used just as much for severe mania, which is how she diagnosed you. A significant number of patients are receiving it now."

"Holy shit." Time for plan B.

Jason proceeds to give me the lay of the land here. "Number one. Your door will always remain open. Two, most importantly, you may never leave this hallway—NEVER. There is a line four feet before the end of the hallway, and that is as far as you go. If you venture beyond that, you will probably be put in restraints and most likely go straight to the ECT treatment room."

I add, "That doesn't sound promising."

He continues, "Three, all meals will be served in your room. You get what they give you, no choice. Four, there is a bathroom, door stays open, no shower, use the sink to wash. Five, you are allowed two visits per day between seven and eight o'clock, up to two people at a time. You must be separated from the visitors by at least four feet, and they cannot enter the hallway. Six, no visiting anyone else in their room. Seven, only one of you in the hallway at a time.

"Follow the rules, and you may get out of here after a couple of days. If not, some are here for a month or more. You have a one-week review meeting with the brass, where they evaluate you. That's five days away."

That's a lot to take in. But I like to find the silver lining in everything. I am now proudly a member of the elite, the special forces of crazies, the craziest of the crazy. Did James Taylor make it here? How about Ray Charles and John Nash? I think not—they made it to MrClean, but not here.

I have one last question. "Can I get coffee in here?"

"Sure," Jason says.

I smile.

My revised plan B is to get the hell out of the untouchables ward that is now the prerequisite to getting the hell out of MrClean. I formulate an unusual plan for me: Follow the rules exactly and put on a charm offensive. Me, a charm offensive? you might ask. Well, yes, I can now be both charming and empathetic—in fact, world-class empathetic. How is that? you might ask.

About two years ago, Lovely Wife told me that although I am wonderful in all aspects, perhaps I could fine-tune my empathy; it needed just a little bit of polish. Of course, I took offense. She proceeded to hand me a book, *Empathy for Dummies* by Dr. Ellen Branch, a professor of psychiatry at Yale University and one of the top psychiatrists in the country.

I intended to speed read it, until . . . I came across the section titled "What If I'm Just Not Empathetic?" That was me.

Her sage advice? "Fake it till you make it."

My thoughts immediately went to one of the greatest movie scenes in history.

"I'll have what she's having," spoken by the lady sitting next to Billy Crystal and Meg Ryan in *When Harry Met Sally*. This line followed Meg's demonstration to a disbelieving Billy that women can, in fact, fake orgasms without men realizing it—a moment brilliantly depicted in this classic film. Little did Meg Ryan know what her faking it might lead her to making it: an actual orgasm.

Dr. Empathy reveals in her book that the latest peer-reviewed research in neurology proves that faking something actually stimulates the neural clusters in the brain that control that "something," which can result in you actually experiencing that something. Hence, you become more empathetic by faking empathy and more orgasmic by faking an orgasm. My best way out is to follow her sage advice—to fake it.

But I'm not trying to have an existential crisis
But I could do without the advice
'Cause it's not easy being me
But it's much harder being a spectacle
My life is upside-down
I'm on the first train out to Crazy Town
There are people worse off,
but they can take it Just gotta fake it 'til I make it

"Fake It 'Til You Make It," Gina Tharin, 2018

Back to the leper ward, and I hear screaming. Seventy-five percent of the words are straight from George Carlin's skit, "Seven Words You Can Never Say on Television." If you haven't seen or heard his act, the words are, in his order, shit, piss, fuck, cunt, cocksucker, motherfucker, and tits. I peer out my door and see the author of this diatribe: a man-boy in his early twenties with rippling muscles, yelling in the hallway. He goes on for at least an hour. Eventually, he retreats to his room, leaving behind what seems like deafening silence. I figure he must have an interesting backstory, so I venture out into the hall and walk to his doorway. He stands up and bolts toward the door.

I warn, “I wouldn’t do that.”

His response is in character: “Why the fucking shit wouldn’t I?”

“Because I’m in the room next to you. I’m in here because I stabbed two motherfuckers in the eye with an ice pick, just because they pissed me off.”

“Did they die?” he asks, seemingly in admiration.

“What the fuck do you think?”

“Now your turn. Why are you in here?”

The rest of the conversation continues with only a few of George Carlin’s words. His name is John. He was abandoned by his parents before he could even remember them. His father had repeatedly beaten his mother in drunken, drug-fueled rages and finally abandoned the family when John was five. He had been working as a landscaper for the last two years after graduating from a local high school. He was addicted to angel dust (PCP), which started out as an anesthetic in the 1950s and was marketed as Sernyl by Parke Davis, now a subsidiary of Pfizer.

He’d attended a party where the host had a large stash of angel dust, which he handed out as party favors. For the nonjunkies, five milligrams of angel dust causes numbness and slurred speech, ten milligrams results in a stupor, fifteen milligrams precipitates paranoia, twenty milligrams leads to extreme violence, twenty-five milligrams triggers psychosis, and thirty milligrams induces a coma. Since it was “free,” he went all in with thirty milligrams and woke up several days later in a hospital, where he heard a nurse whisper, “You’re lucky to be alive, and I really mean, you’re lucky to be alive.”

He was held there for a week then shipped to MrClean and put on what he called “death row.”

When I ask how long he has been here, he says, “Months. This is the first real conversation I’ve had.”

I hear a nurse tell me that dinner is in my room. It is better than expected, some kind of warm meat, potatoes, peas, and a glass of water.

I thank the nurse, and she gives me a surprising, "You're welcome."

No coffee, I guess because it is after 4:00 p.m. I'll just have to figure out how to hoard some later. Just then, I see a cart with a blood pressure gauge and the dreaded blood draw needle. I score a 120/80 blood pressure, pulse 65, and no bitching about the needle. I thank her as she leaves, hoping my much-improved behavior is noted.

Now, who was behind door number two? I look in and see a young girl, maybe eighteen years old. She is sitting on a chair, in her gown, facing sideways to the hallway. She never moves, just stares blankly into the room.

I return to my room, and Jason, the nurse who actually likes me, bounces into the room, smiling, and says, "You've got two guests. Remember to stay behind the line, and you've got just ten minutes."

I exit the room, turn left, and see . . . Lovely Wife and daughter. They are both smiling until John jumps out of his room, looks at my two guests, and lets off a thunderous, rapid-fire recitation of all seven of George Carlin's words.

Their smiles disappear as John starts toward them and explains what he plans to do to them. Immediately, two orderlies rush in, grab him by the arms, and take him to his room, while a nurse follows closely behind with a syringe. Jason walks up to Lovely Wife and daughter and suggests that it might be a good time to go. They decide to stay, as my daughter is returning to New York City later that night. We have an awkward conversation, and they hug me and leave before I can tell them about the no-hugging rule.

I go back to the room, and Jason soon enters. "Sorry about that. John fried his brain, and it's almost impossible to unfry one."

I have a quick flashback to the war on drugs, the ads on TV: two eggs in a frying pan with the caption "This is your brain on drugs." John could have been the poster child.

I pivot the conversation to the occupant across the hall. I motion toward her room and ask, "What's her story?"

"Can't really tell you," Jason replies.

"Okay, let's play a game. I will guess, and if I am right, you nod your head, and if I'm wrong, you shake your head." I go on, "I would bet that she has a history, starting at a very young age, of abuse, probably a member of her family."

Jason nods.

"Recently, she has been seriously beaten," I continue.

Another nod.

"And raped?"

Jason shakes his head.

"But sexually abused?"

A nod.

Holy shit. I stop talking, and Jason leaves.

Not hard to connect these dots. We have a male, whose brain is fried from angel dust, prone to extreme violence, who swears worse than an aircraft carrier full of drunken sailors, less than ten feet from a young female, who has been both beaten and sexually assaulted.

Someone thinks that to put them in close proximity, with open doors, where they can't leave the hall, makes sense—and they call me the crazy one. It's like putting a hungry piranha in a fish tank with a guppy, and an injured one at that.

The more I think about it, and I think about it a lot, the more I believe there are two possible conclusions for their placement of patients. One, they are cutting-edge, brilliant practitioners, whose genius is so blinding that I just can't see it. Or second, it is exactly what it seems, crazy. Exhausted, and perhaps because they've given me a sedative, I fall right to sleep.

CHAPTER 6

"JUST FOLLOW THE RULES"

DAY 4: FRIDAY, AUGUST 3

I wake up early; the clock on the wall reads 5:00 a.m. It's eerily quiet, and I take inventory of my current situation. Even though an unbiased observer, such as Winston Churchill, might describe the key to getting out of here as a "riddle wrapped in a mystery inside an enigma," I'm optimistic about my chances. Just follow the rules. I actually now use "Follow the rules" as my mantra for meditation. Meditation takes two forms: directed and undirected. Directed makes use of a mantra to keep your mind focused and undistracted. Undirected lets your mind go wherever it wants, not something that would be useful for me right now.

However, meditating all the time might seem weird to the powers that be, so I've started to read the book Lovely Wife brought me, *Alice in Wonderland*, rather than the book I crave, the first Harry Potter. She has been warned not to go there. Instead of a theme of good versus evil, it was about an imaginative child growing up. Although I did enjoy the cake with "Eat me" on it that made her grow large, and I certainly did go down a rabbit hole. Oh, well. Stephen Stills had it so right, and I will paraphrase it as "Read the one I'm with," but his lyrics are so much better:

And there's a rose in a fisted glove
And the eagle flies with the dove
And if you can't be with the one you love, honey
Love the one you're with

"Love the One You're With," Stephen Stills, 1970

I still can't figure out who the mystery person is in room 4. They never leave the room, and the door never opens more than a sliver. The nurses enter occasionally, but it remains a mystery to me. Maybe a crazy alien from Area 51? Promptly at 7 a.m., I hear John yelling, "Where's my motherfucking breakfast?" and it arrives within seconds. Somehow, John's consistency is calming to me, and quite entertaining.

After my breakfast, I wander down to John's room and have a quick conversation with surprisingly few of Carlin's words. I tell him I have a rather large property west of Boston, and we use several landscapers.

He asks quietly, "Maybe you could give me a full-time job if I get out of here?"

I say, "Maybe part-time," knowing that it might be a long time before he gets out, like a forever long time.

The rest of the day, I just read *Alice*, and it transports me to a magical world full of curiosity and wonder. My deep dive into Alice is interrupted only by a quick lunch, a check of my vitals, and a bathroom break. I notice the fog lifting a bit, which coincides with the one fewer pill in the little container they handed me and the coffee at breakfast. It looks like they are thinking that I am less of a threat: a good sign.

I remember that the author of Alice used the pseudonym Lewis Carroll, but his real name was Charles Lutwidge Dodgson. No wonder he used a fake name—I would have mercilessly called him "Lut'wedgie" and "Dodgeball." He was a genuine math genius, earning a double first in math and the classics at Oxford, which nobody does. He wrote elaborate solutions to math problems that no one else had solved. He later almost became an Anglican clergyman. He had a stutter and did not seem to have proclivities for women his age. However, he did have a fascination with images of nude young girls. There were rumors, maybe more than rumors, that in 1863 he wished to "marry" eleven-year-old Alice Liddell, from whom the book gets its title.

Now for a short quiz: What did Thomas Edison, Salvador Dali, and Lewis Carroll have in common? Give up? They were all hypnagogians. They realized the creative power of the transitional state between being asleep and awake. Most of us don't even realize we have this superpower. Edison and Dali maximized the effect by holding a small object in their hands, that would then clatter to the floor and wake them up just as they started to doze off. This would go on for hours. It provided the inspiration for Dali's depiction of bending time in his famous painting *The Persistence of Memory* and Edison's receipt of 1,093 patents.

Carroll, on the other hand, would put himself into the "between" state by solving math problems and being aroused by the pencil and pad falling into his lap. Some describe this state as hallucinogenic, and it's also referred to as the *Alice in Wonderland* Syndrome—Google it. Now, to paraphrase Lou Bega's "Mambo No. 5," let's have "a little bit of *Alice* in our tome."

> *"Would you tell me, please, which way I ought to go from here?"*
>
> *"That depends a good deal on where you want to get to," said the Cat. "I don't much care where—" said Alice.*
>
> *"Then it doesn't matter which way you go," said the Cat. "—so long as I get somewhere," Alice added as an explanation.*
>
> *"Oh, you're sure to do that," said the Cat, "if you only walk long enough." "But I don't want to go among mad people," Alice remarked.*
>
> *"Oh, you can't help that," said the Cat. "We're all mad here. I'm mad. You're mad."*
>
> *"How do you know that I'm mad?" said Alice.*
>
> *"You must be," said the Cat, "or you wouldn't have come here."*

The most intriguing part of Alice in Wonderland, for me, is the infamous rabbit hole. Alice's seemingly simple act of falling into a rabbit hole and emerging in Wonderland is more than meets the eye. It's not the destination, but the journey. Geeks find the mathematical backstory interesting, but then again, that's why we were dateless for prom. Any object, including Alice, the object of attention for Carroll, falls down a hole in a predictable path as Newton first described.

So, how did the descent down the rabbit hole play out? Alice followed the rabbit into the infamous rabbit hole. She went from 0 to 22 miles per hour in the first second and hit 60 miles per hour in just 2.7 seconds—faster than 99 percent of the world's Ferraris. After ten seconds, she was plummeting at 220 miles per hour. However, at this point, although her speed continued to increase, her acceleration began to decrease. As you descend through the earth, the gravitational force exerted by the mass of the earth behind you starts to counteract the pull of the mass ahead of you.

Having fun yet? Believe it or not, this is how I pass my time here, doing calculations with edible crayons, made of pure beeswax and available on Amazon. As Alice reached the exact center of the Earth, her acceleration dropped to zero, and her speed peaked at 18,000 miles per hour. She had been falling for twenty-two and a half minutes and had covered 3,963 miles, give or take a couple. She had reached the half-time in her journey, so, it might be fun, like the Super Bowl half-time show, to take a break for a little lighter fare, some differences between British English and American English.

In Britain, Carroll's apparent obsession with young girls earned him the label paedophile, while in America, he would have been labeled a pedophile. The British version is superior. They use "paed," which in Greek means relating to a child. When added to "phile," meaning attracted to, you have someone attracted to a child. While the Americans use "ped," from the Greek *pedo*, which can be mistranslated as "foot," which is clearly more appropriate for someone with a foot fetish.

Halftime was now over. Alice had passed the halfway point, and there was now more earth in her rear than front—think Nicki Minaj or Kim Kardashian. As she continued, gravity was beginning to slow her down, and she was decelerating at an increasing rate, like pushing down on a brake pedal harder and harder.

The deceleration on the way up was the mirror image of the acceleration on the way down. She traveled for an additional twenty-two and a half minutes, covering 3,963 miles. Just as she reached the end of the tunnel, she stopped moving and fell into a heap of sticks on the surface. At this point, I should note that this whole hole scenario is a moot point. In reality, Alice would have burned brighter than Joan of Arc on the stake in 1431, well before she reached the center of the Earth. If Alice had been wearing diamonds, even they would have ignited with the Earth's core being a fiery 10,800 degrees Fahrenheit.

A knock at the door brings me back to my new normal, a hospital named MrClean. For dinner, I am delivered a hot turkey sandwich with gravy; things are looking up.

Even better, Jason, my designated "go to" nurse, has made me a mocha, and he says, with a smile, "Don't tell the boss, and you have a visitor."

I venture out into the "safe zone," four feet from the end of the hallway, and see my neighbor Barry. He and I have done a lot of stupid things together, racing up Mount Washington, a 4,288-foot elevation gain, not once, but ten times. We also "raced" up Mount Fuji, as two of only a handful of gaijin in the three-thousand-person field, mostly stumbling up the 9,842-foot incline.

But wait, there's more. We might have been the only airheads to participate in both the Mount Fuji race and the Pike's Peak Ascent, the latter involving 13.3 miles and 8,000 feet of elevation gain up to the 14,114-foot peak. Barry is also the reason we both ended up climbing the 19,341-foot Mount Kilimanjaro, the highest freestanding mountain in the world. He also sucked me into running with the bulls in Pamplona.

"How's that?" you might ask. More than ten years ago, I asked Barry what was on his bucket list. He claimed to not have one.

However, I pressed him, and he mumbled, "Climbing Kilimanjaro, I guess."

He then countered with, "What's on your bucket list?"

I had to skip over the obvious one (threesome) and finally came to "Running with the bulls in Pamplona."

So, we made a deal: We would cross these two off our lists. I'm not sure if it was a coincidence, but Hemingway had visited both places.

However, Barry was dragging his feet on climbing Kilimanjaro, blaming it on terrorist activity in the area. I gave him a shove by doing it first. I also ran with the bulls later and suggested a little quid pro quo. However, Barry didn't take the bait, probably because he already held an advanced degree in "bull"—a JD degree.

Before Barry can even speak, John rushes out with his usual panoply of maledictions. I use such highbrow language because Barry has an IQ north of 150 with diplomas from very prestigious schools, and he "knows all the best words." He is stunned, but later confesses that the worst part of the experience was catching a glimpse into room 2 and seeing the young girl curled into the fetal position in reaction to John the angel dust guy's outburst.

John charges Barry, but I block the way and hiss something clever like, "Go ahead. Make my day."

Much to everyone's amazement, he retreats quietly back to his room, showing respect for the "ice pick murderer." Things calm down, and I ask Barry to tell the rest of our friends that this Summer Camp is the hottest show in town, and they are welcome to visit.

In a few minutes, Lovely Wife arrives for her daily visit. She informs me that there is a lot happening. My steel fabricator, Paul, urgently needs the sketch for *Newton's Balls*. He has to special-order the stainless steel for the frame, and it will take time to arrive. Stainless steel is tricky to fabricate without ruining the shine. I tell her to have my business partner, Ernie, drop by to pick up the sketch of the balls. He knows the South Boston terrain well and is the perfect person to accomplish the mission of delivering the sketch to the fabrication plant.

Time for a little more about Ernie. He and I have worked together for thirty-five years—more than half my life. Among the hundreds and hundreds of trips we've taken together, two were "around the worlders." We made it in just eight days, during which we spent forty-five hours on an airplane. It was part business, but mostly just for the sheer adventure of it.

One of our stops was Paris, where I took Ernie to see the infamous Crazy Horse show.

Unlike the Moulin Rouge, Crazy Horse was renowned for showcasing completely nude girls. There were nine of them, and they were identical in every way. The opening scene featured all nine of them emerging simultaneously from a wall of fog, created by dropping dry ice in water.

As their identical features were revealed, all at once, Ernie's eyes darted from one to the next, his puritanical upbringing cast aside for a few minutes. He kept murmuring in disbelief, "They're identical. They're identical in every way. Where did they find them?"

I should clarify why I insistently refer to Ernie as my "business" partner. Twenty-five years ago, Ernie and I were traveling on business to San Francisco and enjoyed dinner at a fantastic restaurant.

Toward the end of the meal, the waiter, observing our camaraderie, asked, "You two seem to be having a great time. What brings you to San Francisco?"

I responded, "Ernie and I are partners, doing some sight-seeing and visiting a client."

He followed up with, "How long have you been together? You look like you enjoy each other."

Midway through answering, I realized there was a bit of miscommunication at play. There wasn't much to do but go with it. After all, this was San Francisco, and for the previous twenty-five years, we had spent more time with each other than our "other" spouses. What the hell, we were partners—without benefits, I might add.

On a different note, Lovely Wife complains about Tesla's repeated calls to her. My car is due to be delivered on August 15, just twelve days away. They need details about insurance, the license plate, and most crucially, how I will pay the seventy-five grand.

I assure her, "I'll have instructions ready for you to give my banker, a.k.a. my daughter, tomorrow."

I bid Lovely Wife . . . adieu, once again feeling somewhat Shakespearean, a disposition to which I am often prone. While I'm on the topic of Shakespeare, through my new bipolar lens, I am coming to realize the meaning of Hamlet's famous opening passage in the eponymous play:

To be, or not to be, that is the question:
Whether 'tis nobler in the mind to suffer
The slings and arrows of outrageous fortune,
Or to take Arms against a Sea of troubles,
And by opposing end them: to die, to sleep
No more; and by a sleep, to say we end
The heartache, and the thousand natural shocks
The flesh is heir to.

Hamlet, Shakespeare, 1600

I wonder, could Hamlet have been bipolar? Could Shakespeare have been bipolar? It's plausible. Hamlet is caught in a dilemma of whether to live or die. He is in pain, wrestling with the choice of fight or the ultimate flight: death. Is this suicidal ideation? Ponder no more, as it is time for my own sleep.

CHAPTER 7

"ESCAPE FROM ALCATRAZ"

DAY 5: SATURDAY, AUGUST 4

The next morning, breakfast arrives once again accompanied by caffeinated coffee and a side of cocoa powder.

Jason announces, "You're escaping from Alcatraz; you've set a record for the shortest stay on death row."

Pleasantly surprised, I inquire, "Did you have something to do with that?"

Jason replies with a coy, "Maybe."

I thank him as I gather my crayons and pad and follow him to my room. Several of the other inmates regard me curiously, with a newfound respect that I hadn't noticed before; some even giving me nods of approval.

As I enter my new room, I meet my new, smiling roommate, a rare sight on Ward B South. He gives me a "Hi." After Jason leaves, we have a pleasant chat. He is a student at Brandeis, double majoring in art, specializing in digital media and computer science.

I introduce myself as a fellow aspiring artist, recreating the 1966 *9 Evenings* at the Armory show, a collaboration of art and science.

He responds with an enthusiastic, "Cool. That's what I'm trying to do—not the Armory thing, but the combining art and science part."

I notice his speech is rapid, and he's jumping from one idea to the next. It isn't hard to figure out why he's here. Considering only the most challenging cases end up at MrClean, it isn't mere hypomania—it has to be full-blown mania, officially labeled Bipolar I.

I'm betting this isn't his first rodeo; I'm fairly certain he's been kicked off the bucking bronco several times before. He volunteers that he was just finishing his first year of college when he spiraled into what he calls "warp" drive. For him, everything seemed distorted: Time would alternately slow down and speed up, space both expanding and contracting. He had difficulty sleeping, and he was often surrounded by stupid people.

Until we get to know each other better, we decide to set some ground rules: First, we split the room in half—there is to be no encroaching on the other's territory. No singing, humming, or laughing uncontrollably for no apparent reason.

"How the hell did they allow you to keep your cell phone?" I ask.

He replies, "I've been here before. They let you have a phone if they trust you to not abuse it."

"You don't have a charging cord. How does that work?" I query.

He explains, "They have a charging port near the nurse's area. No cords—they don't want people hanging themselves. They tape over the camera. The HIPAA laws prevent cameras for privacy reasons, which is also why no last names are ever used here."

I approve his cell phone request and propose, "Okay, now let's pinky swear on the ground rules." As we both knew, there is no more solemn contract than that.

Off to lunch with my new roommate, Jonah, and we meet Kerin, who makes three. We arrive early enough to get far up in the queue, ask politely for the turkey sandwich, and head to an unoccupied table. Kerin has been in with Jonah before and vouches for him.

For some reason the word PARTY pops into my head, and I utter the word as I'm thinking it. Kerin and Jonah simultaneously squeal, "YES!"

Oh, well. I have been diagnosed as being chronically "unfiltered," and in this case, it's a good thing. Triggered by either stress or excitement, I simultaneously say what I am thinking. It is similar to Tourette's syndrome, but without the tics. Not always good, especially when you're at a wedding and see an attractive bridesmaid and blurt out, "You're hot," within listening distance of your wife. If I'm quick enough, and I'm pretty quick, I follow up with, "... sweetie," the nickname I use for Lovely Wife, which is usually met with her well-rehearsed eye roll.

We decide that it will be a pizza and ice cream sundae party.

Kerin quickly has it all figured out. "We can't let this leak out, or 'they' will stop it. I'll surreptitiously find out what everyone prefers. We'll start the party tomorrow night after dinner. I know a couple of trustworthy girls, with cell phones, who will help. Everyone will have to be sworn to secrecy, pinky swears all around."

Jonah volunteers to Google and Yelp to find a pizzeria and an ice cream parlor that offer a wide enough selection and will deliver here. During tonight's dinner, the girls will take orders. Since they sometimes have gatherings in the cafeteria after dinner, tomorrow we will set up two tables, an ice cream station, and a pizza table. If the staff asks questions, we will say that we are having a "Bible discussion."

Kerin then says, "Shit. How the hell are we going to pay for it?"

I reply, "Well, I'm pretty good with numbers, as I may have mentioned. Since one of my skills is remembering long strings of numbers, I have memorized all eleven of my credit cards. I've got Visa, Mastercard, Discover, a Bank of America debit card, Costco, Nordstrom ... you name it, I've got it. Oh, yeah, did I mention Amex? Four of them, including, drum roll, a Platinum Card, member since 1976, with no limit."

"Let me repeat that: I can charge as much as I want with no limit. However, I suppose if I go over one million dollars, they might call to confirm." I boast to Jonah, "We can buy a pizzeria or ice cream parlor if we want to."

Jonah exclaims, "Hot damn."

So now, fully energized, Kerin, event planner extraordinaire, is set to turn this dream into a reality. I'm feeling pretty good about this, forgetting about the implications of being sent back to solitary, or worse, the "nuclear option" treatment.

I remember that I still owe a sketch to Paul at Smith & Sons, the stainless-steel fabricator, and head back to my room. I have a prototype of the cradle part of my *Newton's Balls* in the garage. However, the actual weapon-grade product will weigh more than half a ton and have to be anchored with something very heavy.

I am definitely not a structural engineer. However, I did play an engineer my freshman year in college before I switched into a less useful pursuit: math. Suddenly, the long-dormant engineer part of my brain comes alive. Images of Newton and Einstein start to emerge. I will use railroad tracks as the base—they are heavy and cool, and Einstein liked to ride trains since he couldn't drive, and his theory of relativity is best described from the vantage point of someone riding a train.

Now on to a little fun with Newton. His insights led to the toy, Newton's cradle. He didn't make it, but he inspired it. It was actually Simon Prebble, an unremarkable actor, who made the Newton's cradle that we love today in 1967. However, he remained destitute since he couldn't patent it. According to the patent office, he "hadn't improved on Newton." Another guy, seeing an opportunity, stole the idea, and using chrome steel balls, took all the market share. Nevertheless, Prebble wasn't to be denied. He made a giant version for Harrods in London, which was quickly dismantled when it struck a child and knocked him unconscious. Note to self: No children near *Newton's Balls*.

Everything is coming together—Einstein, Newton, and the railroad tracks.

Now, I just need to figure out the exact dimensions of the frame so Paul can begin the fabrication. The good news is that I already know how to get the railroad tracks, located in . . . Newton, Massachusetts.

Kerin, Jonah, and I, all with smirks on our faces, have a quick dinner. Little do the rest of the campers realize that tomorrow night may be the most memorable in the 207-year history of MrClean. Kerin and Jonah will be doing the heavy lifting, and all I'll have to do to become a part of history is remember my fifteen-digit Platinum Amex card number, the expiration date, 10/27, and the four-digit security code, 5124.

I know that Ernie is visiting today from New Hampshire, where he has a house on a lake. That is loon country; they are large, awkward birds. A group of geese is a gaggle; it's a shrewdness of apes, a cauldron of bats, a congregation of alligators, a murder of crows, and—wait for it—an asylum of loons. How fitting from this vantage point.

Ernie arrives one minute early for his visit. He is always on time. He once told me that if you were going to a meeting with ten people, and you were just six minutes late, you would collectively be wasting an hour of time (10 x 6 = 60). In our business, time is money, and people make a lot of money in our business, well over a thousand dollars per hour. Maybe the late one should throw ten Benjamins, the nickname for a hundred-dollar bill, on the table.

It had an effect on me; I was late only once, for a meeting in Mason City, Iowa. I had forgotten to pack a tie on that trip, and in those days, you always wore a tie to a meeting with a client. Luckily, there was a clothing store on the ground floor of their office building, which opened at "9:00 a.m., sharp." My meeting started at 9:00 a.m., sharp, so I would only be slightly late. The next morning, I arrived fifteen minutes early to the building and went to the desk to get my security pass, where the receptionist informed me, "You don't need a security pass in Mason City."

I headed to the door of the store and saw some activity. Ten minutes until meeting time. I waved the clerk over to the door and asked if I could come in early. He pointed to his watch and said, "Nine o'clock sharp, not a second before." I watched my watch. Time seemed to slow down. As my digital watch advanced second by second, I noticed he had a digital watch as well, both of us tuned into the US's primary atomic clock in Boulder, Colorado. At 8:59:59, I hear the door click open.

"What do you need?" he asked.

I answered, "A tie, as fast as I can get one."

He sauntered over, picked out a good-looking tie, and pointed me to the cash register, rang me up, took my credit card, and—wait for it—it cost me 150 bucks.

He smiled, "Hermès. Want it wrapped?"

I didn't have time to argue, but who the hell sells Hermès in Mason City? I grabbed the tie, rushed to the elevator, up to the fourth floor, just enough time to tie the tie.

I walked into the reception area, and the receptionist pointed me to a closed door.

"Go ahead in. The meeting has already started."

The CEO was sitting at the head of the table—CEOs always sit at the head of the table. He tapped his watch and had me sit down at the other end of the table.

"Looks like our guest is a bit late," Mr. Bigshot gloated. I decided I should come clean, told the story of forgetting the tie, and then made a big mistake. I told him I'd paid 150 bucks for the tie.

"What? You paid 150 bucks for that thing. Is that the way you manage our money, overpaying for an ugly tie?"

I did the best I could, but there were snickers all the way around during the rest of the meeting. I heard something like "fancy Nancy" as I was leaving. I lost the account, but did acquire a new tie, a piece-of-shit new tie.

As I was heading back to the airport, it struck me that this was THE Mason City—the place where Buddy Holly, the Big Bopper, and Ritchie Valens died tragically in a 1959 plane crash. The event was memorialized in one of my favorite songs, "American Pie" by Don McLean, released in 1972. Perhaps he was named after this hospital—who knows, life is funny that way. For me it was more like "the day my career died."

Let's return to Ernie and MrClean Insane Asylum. I hand the napkin with my sketch of the frame for *Newton's Balls* to Ernie, who asks, "Do I have something on my face?"

Ernie can be a funny guy, and I'm not entirely sure if he's joking. Nonetheless, I give him the benefit of the doubt. I point to the diagram on the napkin. He can be a tough critic, but he says he likes it. I inform him that Paul at Smith & Sons in South Boston is expecting him and give him the name and address of the place. He says he's got it covered; he knows "Southie," and will be there when they open at 7:00 a.m. sharp. I have no doubt he will.

Ernie departs just as Lovely Wife walks in. She asks how things are going. Am I getting stressed out? How am I sleeping?

I reassure her, "I've got it under control, no problem."

She gives me a "Sure you do" smile.

The real answer is, "Of course I'm stressed out. I'm in a fucking insane asylum with no easy way out."

Lovely Wife seems somewhat relieved and gently suggests, "Please don't do anything that will upset the doctors."

I decide to keep the details of the imminent "party to end all parties" to myself, considering it might not be well-received. However, I do ask her to bring me a particular set of clothes for my one-week review meeting on Monday: my black power outfit.

This outfit is intended to demonstrate that I am not some quivering soul, beaten down by the medications that are meant to suppress my spirit, my essence. Rather than "fuck-me clothes," they are "fuck-you clothes."

As she's leaving, she casually mentions, "One more thing. GB and I have moved the show from September 5 to October 19. It's nonnegotiable." She turns and utters a quick "adieu" before I can launch into my "woe is me" routine.

I rapidly cycle through the five stages of grief: denial, anger, bargaining, depression, and acceptance. She and GB are, of course, right. Rushing the show would result in a catastrophe akin to Samuel Beckett's *Waiting for Godot*—a no-show.

Back in my room, Jonah excitedly waves a piece of paper. "I found them! I found them! I got a pizzeria and ice cream place that have what we need. Sweetheart has the best selection of ice cream in the Boston area, with every type of topping, including red and black licorice. It has a 4.7 rating on Google with fifty-one reviews. Belmont Pizza, with a 4.5 rating on Google from 206 reviews, has toppings that range from asparagus to ziti. Get it? A to Z."

I ask, "Do they accept Amex, and did they confirm delivery to MrClean?"

"Yes, and yes," Jonah confirms.

"Great job, Jonah."

He beams with pride.

"Big day tomorrow. Let's try to get some sleep," knowing that neither Jonah nor I will get a single wink.

CHAPTER 8

"LET'S GET THE PARTY STARTED"

DAY 6: SUNDAY, AUGUST 5

We wake up at 6:30 a.m. and take turns for our supervised bathroom time. I'm ecstatic that I am permitted to use the safety razor. However, I still have to go to the locked cabinet and ask one of the nurses to retrieve it for me, and I must return it posthaste.

Shaving doesn't go smoothly. The cheap plastic razors, likely costing the hospital twenty-five bucks each, struggle against my six-day stubble. The high-quality shaving cream somewhat makes up for it. Note to self: Sneak as many cans home as I can. Breakfast consists of a double dose of my custom mocha, or "doppio," as the Italians say.

I still haven't explored the rest of the ward. So, I decide to meet my fellow inmates on a walkabout. Almost immediately, a young man, who could easily be mistaken for Hercules, approaches me.

"I need your help. I'm scheduled for ECT tomorrow morning, and I'm kind of afraid. Will I be all right?" he asks.

I'm shocked. Shock therapy? Not just shocked—I am high-voltage shocked, and disgusted and goddamn angry, really angry, pissed-off angry. How could this be? This is insane. I know Jason had mentioned it earlier, but I thought he was just trying to scare me. Are they really still giving shock therapy to victims—I mean, patients? I was certain that ECT was discontinued after the public uproar following the release of Ken Kesey's influential novel *One Flew over the Cuckoo's Nest* in 1962. Its adaptation into a movie in 1975, featuring Oscar-winning performances by Jack Nicholson as a patient and Louise Fletcher's chilling portrayal of his nemesis, Nurse Ratched, fueled the public opposition. They are regarded as two of the finest performances in movie history.

In a nutshell, the story revolves around Nicholson's character, McMurphy, who feigns insanity to avoid hard labor for various crimes, including statutory rape. However, once inside the asylum, he provokes Nurse Ratched by leading a revolt against her authority. ECT is her prime weapon—not to aid him, but to incapacitate him, ensuring he bends to her will.

To comfort Hercules, I reassure him, "Sure. Everything's going to be all right."

The staff has informed him that the treatment will significantly improve his condition.

Despite hearing echoes of "Cuckoo, cuckoo, cuckoo" over and over in my head, it seems better at this point to ease his anxiety and distract him from the impending procedure. I ask him about how he ended up in Summer Camp. His name is Ben, twenty years old and in his final year of college.

Ben is an elite wrestler, an undefeated NCAA Division 1 champion for three straight years in the 197-pound class. He'd suffered a dislocated shoulder, which forced him to take a break from his extensive training about six months earlier. He became depressed. He underwent all the usual treatments, starting with cognitive behavioral therapy, which provided no help. He cycled through multiple psychiatrists and antidepressants; vilazodone, a serotonin booster, Prozac, a selective serotonin reuptake inhibitor (SSRI), fluoxetine, another SSRI with a different approach to limiting the reuptake of serotonin, and so on. Since nothing worked, he got the diagnosis of "treatment-resistant depression." In other words, "We don't have a clue how to help."

His experience isn't unique. We are finding out that it's fairly common among elite athletes who dedicate long hours to training. The most notable example is Michael Phelps, the swimmer who won twenty-three gold medals—the most in modern Olympic history—over the span of twelve years. Phelps trained for more than five hours a day, racking up more than twenty thousand hours during his career, perhaps more than any other person.

However, Phelps had a severe, undiagnosed case of depression, which he self-medicated with rigorous exercise. Prolonged physical activity triggers your body to release both endorphins and dopamine. Endorphins cause the "runner's high" many athletes experience. However, extensive exercise also causes a buildup of dopamine. This powerful neurotransmitter induces euphoria and has effects similar to those of the antidepressants called norepinephrine and dopamine reuptake inhibitors.

When Michael Phelps stopped producing large quantities of dopamine, he experienced withdrawal and plunged into severe depression.

I ask Ben, "What's your go-to pinning move?"

"The drop cradle. You know what that is?" he asks.

"Indeed, I do. It begins with the referee's position. The guy on top applies a cross-face, threads his other arm through his opponent's legs, locks arms, flips him onto his back, and three seconds later, the ref slams his hand to the mat. PIN! It's effective 95 percent of the time."

"Holy shit. You wrestled?" asks Ben.

"Yeah, but I sucked. My career ended in eighth grade when I tried a Granby Roll." (It's like a somersault, with the other wrestler holding your wrist.) "My arm, with a distinct cracking sound, bent the wrong way and just hung limp. I told the ref that it didn't hurt, but I ended up in an ambulance. The ER doctor claimed it was the worst dislocation he'd ever seen.

I said, "At least it isn't broken."

He laughed and responded, "You'd be much better off if it were just broken. You'll be lucky if you ever straighten your arm again."

My arm was in a sling for a year. The only upside was that I looked so pathetic and helpless that some of the cute girls offered to carry my books. That's when I learned a great life lesson: Girls like it when a guy is vulnerable. To this day, my arm doesn't straighten.

There are approaches than "seem" to improve "some" bipolar patients. Emphasis on "seem" and "some" because it's been observed that a meaningful percentage of untreated patients go into remission on their own. No one knows why.

Let's move on to the scientific testing of bipolar drugs, also known as drug trials.

Thousands of these trials have been conducted, and the gold standard is the double-blind test. In such trials, patients are divided into two groups: one receives the actual drug, and the other a placebo, a fancy word for something that looks like the drug but is inert. In the old days, they called it a "sugar pill." The doctor administering the drug is also "blind," meaning neither the patient nor the doctor knows real from fake.

At the conclusion of the trial, the envelope with the results is opened. The anxiety must be similar to opening the envelope with your college board scores. If it's good, you're set for life; if bad, you hear a toilet-flushing sound. The big reveal, virtually none of the drugs outperform the placebo. Billions have been spent on these studies with positive results as elusive as alchemist's gold.

The vast majority of these studies have been funded by the drug companies hoping to sell their miracle drug to people who, by their nature, may be crazy enough to buy them. The best part for the drug companies is that once you find a drug that you can tolerate, you are on it for life, whether it "works" or not.

Once again, here comes my inner math geek. A fraction of the trials seems to show a meaningful positive result—the nerds call it a statistically significant result—where they are 95 percent confident the result isn't due to chance. What they don't tell you is that conclusion is most likely wrong.

More than forty years ago, I learned about a key statistical concept called "the joint test of significance." Judgments on drugs are usually made based on published trials in fancy medical journals, where the articles are peer-reviewed, to ensure no errors or even outright fraud. The peers, usually called referees, give a nod that is equivalent to the *Good Housekeeping* Seal of approval.

However, there is a dirty secret: Out of one hundred trials, maybe five show statistically significant results, where the drug being tested is more effective than a placebo. The remaining ninety-five, which show no statistically significant effect, go unpublished. The pharmaceutical companies fund most of the research and don't submit the failures for publication. They are the invisible majority. The five successes are the only ones we see, and when submitted to the FDA, the drugs often get approved. However, the powerful "joint test of significance" now comes into play. Collectively, out of a hundred trials, if the results were random, we would expect to observe five "statistically significant" trials. If the hidden ninety-five were exposed, the "significant" five would be revealed to be insignificant. It's a scam.

Now for the good news. It is hard for a drug to beat a placebo since the latter is a powerful and efficacious drug, with NO side effects. Thousands of trials have demonstrated that a placebo significantly outperforms nothing at all. Patients often improve simply because they believe a drug will help them—the infamous "placebo effect." However, a placebo can't be prescribed because it is not recognized as a "drug." So, we're left with a dilemma.

Actual drugs, which often have serious side effects and come with a high cost, will help patients, primarily because the patients believe they will. And, since placebos are banned as medication, then the five out of a hundred drugs that sneak through the trials, if only because they evoke the placebo effect, are better than nothing.

Perhaps in the not-too-distant future, someone will submit a trial for a new drug, Obecalp. Perhaps, just by chance, it will perform well enough in the clinical trials to get FDA approval. Patients will then pick it up at their local pharmacy, where the pharmacist will give detailed instructions on how to take this new, powerful drug. Miraculously, most patients will improve, with no side effects. Of course, I will have the patent on this drug, Obecalp—which is placebo spelled backward. I just love a good emordnilap.

Back to the "some" in the "seem" to make "some" patients "better" mentioned earlier.

There's a significant subgroup of patients suffering from depression who don't respond to any treatment and are classified as having treatment-resistant depression (TRD). Nothing, not even the kitchen sink, seems to help. Ben has TRD, and that's why he is scheduled in one hour to get ECT. The medical community currently refers to it as the "gold standard." However, I consider it the "iron pyrite standard." For the non-geologists, iron pyrite is fool's gold. Read on.

Now, a brief primer on ECT. At this point I hear some grumbling: Why listen to him? He's not a doctor. That is true; however, maybe that's the point. Sometimes it is better to be curious rather than degreed. This is what those prescribing ECT don't tell you, nor is it mentioned very often in the peer-reviewed, gold-standard articles published in the fancy medical journals. Paul Harvey, the legendary radio personality whose show was on for four decades, called it "the rest of the story." In 1934, a Hungarian doctor, Ladislas Meduna, saw marginally positive results in a patient with psychosis by inducing a seizure with a very high dose of Metrazol, a stimulant. In medicine, where everything needs a fancy name, this procedure was called pharmacologic convulsive therapy (PCT).

However, PCT had a major side effect—it caused such violent convulsions that patients often ended up with self-induced vertebral fractures, in addition to the fear of a horrendous death. The medical community began to ponder if there might be a less harmful way to induce a seizure. It is told that a few years later, Ugo Cerletti happened to be shopping at a butcher's shop when he observed the butcher deliver an electrical shock to a pig about to be slaughtered.

Remarkably, the pig experienced the exact type of seizure Cerletti sought, rendering it docile and easy to slaughter. This observation led Cerletti to the idea for a new procedure, which he named electroshock therapy.

Upon returning to his lab, Cerletti gathered some electrodes and a generator and set to work. An unsuspecting stray dog in the street happened by his office and became the first "volunteer." Cerletti inexplicably attached one electrode to the dog's mouth and the other into the dog's anus. You read that right, anus. You can't make this stuff up. Guess what happened? The dog died an excruciating death, its cries echoing for miles away.

The electrode up the ass thing brings to mind another "gold-standard" procedure from the Middle Ages: Shoving a red-hot poker up someone's ass was considered an exceptionally brutal form of torture, the best. On September 21, 1327, it was reported that King Edward II was murdered in this manner. His wife and her lover were blamed. Allegedly, his screams could be heard from miles away.

Unfazed by the death of the first dog, Cerletti persisted, tweaking his approach until he recalled the butcher's technique. When he attached both electrodes to a dog's head instead, with the electric current bypassing the heart, he achieved the desired seizure with a lower probability of death.

The next step was to test the method on a human guinea pig: a homeless man with schizophrenia, who was seen wandering the streets much like the stray dogs. Cerletti's colleagues apprehended the vagrant and brought him to the lab. Without anesthesia, they connected the electrodes to his head. When only a minor spasm but no seizure occurred, Cerletti raised the voltage to ninety volts. Still no seizure. Then one hundred volts. Nothing. They continued until they succeeded. They were quick to note that the "volunteer" didn't die, but he couldn't remember anything—especially his pleas of "Stop, stop, you are killing me!" before he passed out in a convulsive fit.

Modern ECT procedures are somewhat less harsh. Patients receive anesthesia, so they don't recall the trauma, and the doctors don't have to endure their screams. Another advancement in ECT treatment is that patients now are administered muscle relaxants to prevent whiplash and other bodily damage caused by thrashing around while convulsing.

This replaced the bite block that was used to prevent patients from breaking their teeth during a seizure. You've probably seen them used in old Western movies when the town doctor, after giving the loser of a gunfight a big swig of booze, would insert a bite block into his mouth before removing a bullet with pliers. The doctors are also getting support—they are now provided with training to cope with post-traumatic stress disorder (PTSD). ECT can be traumatic for the giver as well as the receiver.

I tell Ben I'll visit him before his treatment tomorrow and head to the cafeteria a bit early. As the doors open, I'm third in line for lunch, with Kerin just behind me. She whispers that she wants to give me an update on tonight's party and asks me to meet her in the activity room in about thirty minutes. We wolf down lunch and head to our rooms to get ready for our meeting.

In the activity room, Kerin is sitting on a sofa at the back and signals me to join her.

"It's all set," she says with a spark of joy in her eyes.

I give her a puzzled look as she elaborates.

"The party is all set. We have everyone's order for pizza and ice cream—from the type and number of pizza slices to ice cream flavors, the number of scoops, choice of sauce, and the preferred type of sprinkles." We'll even sneak some treats to those on death row.

I add, "Don't forget the whipped cream."

Her quick retort comes, “Everyone likes whipped cream, even the lactose intolerants.” She definitely has that right.

She outlines the rest of the plan: Jonah will place the orders at 7:15 p.m. for delivery at 7:45 p.m., just as visiting hour ends. Meanwhile the Bible discussion is set to begin in the reserved dining room at 8:00 p.m. My job is to manage the payment. I need to stand next to Jonah, who will hand me his phone when it is time to make the charge. Looks like things are under control. This reminds me of George Peppard’s character, Colonel John “Hannibal” Smith, from the classic TV show *A-Team*. He often quipped to Mr. T., “I love it when a plan comes together,” and this plan is together.

However, part of our plan is to keep things quiet; loose lips sink parties. Anticipating my concern, Kerin assures me that no one will spill the beans because everyone loves the idea and hates the wardens.

I ask somewhat incredulously, “Even Slugger?” This is the nickname I’ve given to the woman who beat the shit out of me.

“Especially her,” Kerin replies. “She actually likes you.”

Feeling pretty good, I head back to my room, stopping at the cafeteria to grab my custom mocha and two “high-test” cups of coffee and cocoa mixes for my post-4 p.m. caffeine fix. Anticipating a long day, I decide to double up. Back in the room, I am beaming, high-fiving the air. I can’t wait for this party to get started.

Jonah struts in, as excited as I am. He breaks out his meticulous lists, detailing each guest’s preferences. For instance, the pizza order list totals sixty-two slices: twenty pepperoni, sixteen cheese, eight mushroom, eight veggie, eight meat, and two Hawaiian. Given that each pizza has eight slices, that works out to two and a half pepperoni pies, two cheese, one each of mushroom, veggie, and meat, and half a Hawaiian pizza since that’s the smallest quantity we can order.

He boasts, “The pizzeria is also giving us oregano and garlic on the side, to add to taste. They’re also giving us the hospital discount of five bucks per pie and waiving the tax. So, for eight pizzas, that’s a grand total of—wait for it—exactly forty dollars.”

I notice that Jonah has picked up my intentionally annoying “wait for it” and am pleased.

"Shit," Jonah says. "I forgot you."

"No problem—I'll take the two extra slices of the Hawaiian, although I think it's weird putting pineapple on pizza," I say.

He then takes out his equally detailed ice cream sundae list and adds my choice: vanilla, a no-brainer, three scoops. He notes that everyone wants three scoops, so that makes sixty-six scoops in total: forty vanilla, twelve chocolate, eight strawberry, and six chocolate chip. With eight scoops in a quart, and four scoops a pint, we need five quarts of vanilla, one quart and one pint of chocolate, and one quart each of strawberry and chocolate chip. We're not too worried about the extra two scoops of chocolate chip; someone will eat it. Jonah, once again, receives the hospital special: four bucks a quart, they throw in the pint for free, and again, no sales tax, for a grand total of—let's skip the "wait for it"—thirty-six buckaroos.

The best part? They're also giving us a quart of fudge sauce, a pint each of caramel and strawberry sauce, a cup each of chocolate and rainbow sprinkles, and a whole gallon of fresh whipped cream. This whole shindig will set us back a whopping seventy-six dollars.

"Excellent work, Jonah," I say, and give him a thumbs-up—make that a double thumbs-up.

A sudden realization hits me: I am not leading the existential fight of good versus evil that I once thought I was. I am not Harry Potter, supported by the usual cast of characters with moai and *Newton's Balls* thrown in, destined to fight Voldemort, the epitome of evil, in a showdown to determine the fate of humankind. Instead, I'm leading a different battle. I'm leading this band of misfits against the tyranny of a deeply entrenched medical system, where fear of malpractice suits trumps compassionate care. I do feel the weight of the ward on my shoulders—not quite Atlas-like, but perhaps Wilt Chamberlain–like, who carried the Philadelphia 76ers on his broad shoulders for many years. "Wilt the Stilt" actually scored a hundred points in one game. I listened to it on my transistor radio, under the covers as it was past my bedtime. No one has come close since then.

I snap back to reality as it's time for dinner. Jonah and I depart, checking Kerin's room on the way. However, it is empty. She's already queued up—first in line, I'm two, and Jonah's three. I hate being a number two, so I surreptitiously swap places with Jonah. As the other patients file in, they all look over, giving a wave, a smile, a thumbs-up, or some combination of the three.

Jason, the good nurse, walks over, informing us that the cafeteria is all ours for the Bible study group after dinner. With a smile, he assures us that he will make sure that we aren't disturbed. Yes, there is a God. Let the games begin. Lovely Wife will soon arrive, and I want to appear well-groomed to make her feel that everything is moving in the right direction. I am now allowed to shave, and I have the nurse retrieve a disposable razor from lockdown. I grab the small can of shaving cream that they actually let you keep, and I meet him in the bathroom.

Shaving with a cheap disposable razor is not without its challenges, particularly around the nose. A fresh blade is always dangerous, making it ridiculously easy to cut yourself, and razor cuts bleed profusely. Although the bleeding usually stops within five to ten minutes, it leaves a telltale bloody ridge. Not a good look, and I definitely want to look good tonight, not just for Lovely Wife, but for the most epic party ever.

Surprisingly, Lovely Wife shows up promptly at 7:00 p.m. with a bag containing my power outfit for tomorrow. I check to make sure everything is there. She asks how it's going. I tell her everything is going well, and I am looking forward to tomorrow's meeting at 11:00 a.m.

"Ten thirty a.m. The meeting's at 10:30," she corrects me.

"Oh, yeah, 10:30 a.m. I can't wait," I respond.

She knows me well. I suspect that she suspects something's up.

I deflect to, "I have to get ready for the 'Bible meeting.' I'm leading the discussion."

She shakes her head and walks away.

Once the meal is finished, several diners morph into an efficient crew. Some arrange the tables and chairs into the pizza and ice cream sundae stations, while others decorate the room with crepe paper streamers made in art class. A young girl, who just finished her first year at MIT, and apparently a tech genius, is setting up her iPhone to play music.

Suddenly, the room fills with sound.

I ask, "How the hell did you do that?"

She responds, "Just a few hacks; adjust the EQ equalizer, turn off the headphone safety, but most importantly place the cell phone in a round bowl, with the speakers facing down. The sound waves bounce off the sides into the air."

Amazing.

"What is your playlist?" I query.

She smiles. "I Googled 'best party songs' and compiled the top songs."

As attendees begin to trickle into the cafeteria, buzzing with anticipation for the party to begin, DJ MIT decides to provide some background music and tests the sound system. She plays James Taylor's "Fire and Rain" as the trickle turns into a stream. This is THE Sweet Baby James who was treated for depression at MrClean. His lyrics suggest that he might have actually been bipolar, with lines like "I've seen summer days I thought would never end," and "I've seen lonely times when I could not find a friend." We keep this song on repeat until everyone finishes eating and is ready to dance.

I've seen fire and I've seen rain
I've seen sunny days that I thought would never end
I've seen lonely times when I could not find a friend
But I always thought that I'd see you again . . .
Been walking my mind to an easy time
My back turned towards the sun
Lord knows, when the cold wind blows
It'll turn your head around
Well, there's hours of time on the telephone line
To talk about things to come
Sweet dreams and flying machines
in pieces on the ground . . .
I've seen lonely times when I could not find a friend
But I always thought that I'd see you again

"Fire and Rain," James Taylor, 1970

Jason peeks in and announces there are two deliveries for Jonah. At this point, I'm pretty sure that Jason has figured everything out. Jonah heads to the door and is met with a stack of pizza boxes about a foot and a half tall and two large freezer bags containing the ice cream and the whipped cream. A separate bag contains the toppings.

At 8:00 p.m. sharp, the doors open, and the rest of the partiers enter and descend on the goods. Everyone moves deliberately, without rushing. We have an hour for the party—I mean, Bible study group. To be fair, in John 16:24, Jesus said, "Ask and you shall receive," and it won't take long for everyone to receive exactly what they asked for; a Bible lesson well-learned.

Surveying the scene, I notice everyone begins with the pizza. I'm struck by the variety of ways to eat pizza. The most popular method is the "hand" technique, picking up the pizza slice and eating from the pointed bottom end. Many, including myself, employ the "folder" technique, where the pizza is folded in half and eaten from the bottom. Kerin, along with most of the women, opts for the "knife and fork" style.

One partygoer adopts John Travolta's "stack and shove" method, as seen in *Saturday Night Fever*, 1977—stacking one slice of Hawaiian on top of another, then shoving both into his mouth. I can't help but smile when I realize it's Ben channeling Travolta—welcome to the party! The final three techniques are the "upside down," the "backward," and the "topping remover," which I find perplexing. What's the point of ordering a pizza and taking off the toppings? Let them eat bread.

The crowd quickly transitions to the ice cream sundae station. Three volunteers scoop out the chosen flavors for each of the partygoers, who then move to the toppings. Some carefully layer hot fudge, followed by rainbow sprinkles, topped with a dollop of whipped cream.

Others simply heap on everything, then squish it all together. Everyone indulges in the whipped cream.

All enjoy their pizza and ice cream. The pizza is flat-out amazing and, literally, finger-licking good—except for the "knife and forkers," for whom it is, only figuratively, finger-licking good.

It's fortunate that we have plenty of paper towels for people to wipe off their hands and faces. We're all so heavily medicated and zapped by ECT that we are, no sugarcoating it, slobs. The crowd is breaking into smaller groups, and all I can see on their faces is joy. Let me repeat, since this is crucial—pure joy in a mental institution where over half the patients are not merely depressed, but treatment-resistant depressed.

Joy is a powerful word. In the spirit of this being a Bible group meeting, I'll mention that the words *joy*, *joyful*, and *rejoice* appear 430 times in the Bible. My favorite, Isaiah 55:12: "You will go out in joy and be led forth in peace; the mountains and hills will burst into song before you, and all the trees of the field will clap their hands." I have to admit it—I feel the joy as well. If the price I have to pay for this epic party is another week in here, then so be it. I will deal with that tomorrow. Time to crank it up.

"DJ MIT, cue up the first song."

And so, it begins.

"Get the Party Started" is sung by someone who grew up just a few miles from me, Pink. The guests are still mostly in small groups, standing silently, others engaged in quiet conversation. I notice Slugger has made the scene and is standing alone in a corner fidgeting, but not to the music. She seems to be mumbling—she's always mumbling, always complaining. Ben is standing in the doorway. I suspect he might be contemplating an early exit, so I motion him over and encourage him to stay.

"Hang around for a while. Things are about to get interesting."

He nods.

A couple of the girls start to sway a bit to the music, and I'm relieved that at least this won't be a total bust. DJ MIT has obviously done this before, as she transitions seamlessly into Whitney Houston's "I Want to Dance with Somebody" and Donna Summer's "I Feel Love." With Kerin's encouragement, a few more partygoers venture onto the dance floor.

However, with classics like these, I was hoping for more. Michael Jackson's "Thriller" does ignite the crowd. About half the group moves to the center of the floor, actually moving to the music.

The first few songs elicit little reaction from the group, then it happens: the Village People's "YMCA," perhaps the greatest party song ever, hits the air. It is played at every wedding, bar mitzvah, sixty-fifth birthday party, and gay funeral. I think that if I had to choose to be one of the People, I'd be the guy with the tool belt, going by the handle "The Hammer."

Miraculously, Ben and—wait for it—Slugger join the fun. Their arms are raised, spelling out Y-M-C-A, although the arm movements are a bit out of sync with the music. Utter delight radiates from everyone's face. More incredibly, when the song ends and "Last Dance" begins to play, Slugger walks over.

I cringe a bit, and she hits me with, "Wanna dance?"

Last dance
Last chance for love
Yes, it's my last chance
For romance tonight
So let's dance the last dance
Let's dance the last dance
Let's dance the last dance tonight

"Last Dance," Donna Summer, 1978

Jason peeks in and holds up ten fingers, signaling that we'd better be back in our rooms in ten minutes. I figure the cleanup will be quicker with five people instead of eighteen. I ask for volunteers; everyone raises their hand. I select Kerin and Jonah, knowing they will do a great job, as well as two others who are waving their hands energetically. Their enthusiasm reminds me of Arnold Horshack in *Welcome Back, Kotter*, 1975. Whenever Mr. Kotter, a teacher played by Gabe Kaplan, would ask his class a question, Arnold would frantically wave his hand and yell, "OOH, OOH, OOH," hoping to get called. It usually worked.

Cleanup is swift, and we finish with two minutes to spare. The two volunteers, their task completed, leave. Kerin and Jonah ask me to stay, promising to keep it short.

Jonah begins, "This is the first time in a long time that someone actually trusted me to do an important job. You not only gave me one, but you also told me I did a great job. I actually do believe I did a great job. Once again, I feel that I can meet the expectations of becoming successful."

Kerin adds, "Thank you. You've shown me something that I had forgotten: joy. That's the best reason to go on living. Everyone else just tries to keep me from dying."

At his point, I gasp and begin to cry. Jonah and Kerin look perplexed. I tell them that they are very wise for those so young. They have distilled the problem with the mental health care system into just a few insightful words. Patients do not have to be on a lifetime of powerful meds—they just need someone to trust them and show them joy. Preventing death is not living.

We say our goodbyes, and I head to my room. Tomorrow, I'm going to face the music. However, today I feel contentment. As soon as my head hits the pillow, I'm out, maybe even on the way down.

CHAPTER 9

"WHAT'S THE DIFFERENCE BETWEEN MY STAY HERE AND CHARLES MANSON'S?"

DAY 7: MONDAY, AUGUST 6

I decide to skip breakfast and meet Jason in the bathroom.

He smiles and says, "Great party. First one we've ever had."

I thank him.

Jason goes on, "Dr. Ratched knows about the party. She's livid. There's no way you're getting out anytime soon. Just watch it. ECT may still be on the table."

I do wonder if one doctor can unilaterally prescribe the treatment. You would think that there would have to be some kind of appeals process. However, I have learned that MrClean, along with the Mayo Clinic and Johns Hopkins, employs the technique more than any other medical facility. So, I'm glad that I have a couple of tricks up my sleeve.

"One way or another, that's not happening to me."

It suddenly hits me that my nemesis, Dr. Ratched, and I have not yet met. So far, she has been a theoretical construct, and it's hard to deal with a concept. However, I'm pretty good at dealing with adversaries, and I do consider her that. I know how to play mind games, even under the influence of their drugs, which fight one of the good aspects of mania, the creative part of the brain that can be mischievous. Caffeine will also help me remain sharp.

Another help will be that Dr. Empathy, my friend and teacher, will be visiting after our meeting to see how things went.

Bipolars tend to think differently, often in nonlinear ways. This ability allows us to solve problems, but also envision opportunities that nobody else can see. We not only think outside the box, but we also don't even know the notion of a box. Interestingly, these "innovators" never for a second doubt they will succeed. Their "delusions of grandeur" sometimes allow them to see what others cannot. A future that does not yet exist.

Elon Musk, the poster-child wizard, pioneers innovative ways to drive cars and fly rockets. Teddy Roosevelt, another famous recipient of the "gift," led the Rough Riders to the top of San Juan Hill in Cuba on July 1, 1898. This audacious act effectively ended the Spanish-American War, as well as Spain's rule as the most powerful empire in the world. Every one of his advisers deemed it impossible, even insane. He ignored them, leading the charge on his horse. His men followed.

Picasso and Hemingway, arguably the greatest artist and writer of the twentieth century, respectively, were most likely bipolar. They revolutionized their respective fields. So, were they crazy?

Yeah, crazy talented. I'd argue that almost every innovation that has made this world better has been done by the "crazies" with their "gifts." Fewer than 0.0001 percent of the world's population, the proverbial one in a million, do almost all the heavy lifting.

Enough of the self-pep talk. I do my usual routine, wash my hands, brush my teeth, hit the toilet, shower—headfirst, then working my way down—towel off, shave, and head back to my room. I grab a pair of PJs on my way back to the room. Soon, I'll be donning an outfit suitable for the fashionista that I am. Shit, I almost forgot: I promised Ben, a.k.a. Hercules, that I'd be there for him before his ECT treatment. I go off to find him.

Ben did show up at the party, but he was clearly anxious about the impending treatment. Despite this, he managed to wolf down his pizza and scarf down the ice cream sundae. He even swayed a bit to the music. I see Ben outside an unmarked door I hadn't noticed before. An unmarked door in a hospital usually means that something bad is on the other side. I suppose a sign reading "Danger: High Voltage" wouldn't be a good look.

Before he asks, I offer my requisite placebo comment: "It's going to be all right. The treatment will help you get better."

He asks me to wait outside the procedure room until he returns.

"I'll be here," I assure him.

He's led through the door, and I ask a nurse how long it will take.

She replies, "About an hour."

After five minutes, I grow restless and decide to pace the halls of the ward. I calculate that I've walked about two miles when I see Ben being escorted back to his room. This world-class athlete has to be held up as he staggers toward his room and is slowly lowered into a chair in the hallway.

The nurse suggests, "Give him a few minutes. He's just tired from the treatment."

I grab another chair and sit next to him. His head is slumped, gently swaying side to side. He's clearly disoriented, seemingly unsure of where he is, or even who I am or he is.

He mumbles something like, "How did I do?" I presume he is talking about a wrestling match.

I reassure him that he won the match and remains the NCAA champ. He nods.

Once again, I am both angry and confused. What am I missing? The doctors at the most prestigious mental hospital in the country think that what seems to me to be a cruel procedure is the best that can be done. Where is the evidence? It seems like I'm living in an alternative universe. It doesn't make any sense. We have to be able to do better. The doctors here are smart and want to help the patients—they even believe shock treatments are effective. However, they can't be happy with the status quo.

After about half an hour, he starts to look a little more with it. I ask him if he knows where he is.

He manages, "In the hospital."

I ask, "Do you know what just happened?"

He admits, "Not really."

I follow up with, "How do you feel?"

He shakes his head, and says, "I kind of feel like throwing up, I have a bad headache, and I'm tired and confused."

I look at my watch and realize I have to go. I assure him that I'll check in on him later.

Back to my room. I don't have much time. Fortunately, I have everything laid out on the bed. I start with the slick black Uniqlo underwear, followed by my black Theory pants, then my black Bugatchi shirt. I sit down and put on my black Smartwool liner socks, then slide into my "dead guy" black Prada loafers. (I got a great deal on them since I bought them from the estate of someone who was wearing them when he died.) Finally, I slip into my black Zegna sport coat, and I've transformed into a sartorial god.

Lovely Wife arrives at 10:25, surprisingly early. We gather outside the conference room. At exactly 10:30 a.m., Jason, I really like that guy, invites us to go in. There are seven self-important-looking doctors and a social worker sitting around the table. I see at the head of table someone I presume is Dr. Ratched, our first face-to-face. Just a quick aside: I have found that truly great leaders never sit at the head of the table. They are secure enough that they don't need to intimidate others with that minor-league stunt.

I may not be the physically strongest one in a fight, but I seldom lose a battle of wits. Dr. Ratched has already betrayed her insecurity. I thrive in chaos; I am nimble, I adapt quickly, and I use the fog of uncertainty I create to my advantage. It's time to create some chaos and turn the floor into quicksand.

Lovely Wife and I settle at the opposite end of the table.

With a stern look on her face, Dr. Ratched begins, "Why are you dressed like that?"

I laugh and retort, "I'm sure you're aware, but if you wish, I'll spell it out for you." I continue, "I'm simply leveling the playing field. You're dressed up to show your superior status. If I showed up in PJs, you'd categorize me as a mere patient in critical need of your assistance. It's true that first impressions are everything."

"Why is that?" she asks condescendingly, as if it's the ultimate "gotcha" question.

"Because of confirmation bias and cognitive dissonance. Once someone forms a first impression, it becomes virtually impossible to change it. All subsequent information is filtered through this initial impression, and only the facts that support it are allowed to pass through. Essentially, I would be dismissed within the first few seconds. I've leveled the attire playing field now. I think I look pretty good. Moreover, I've succeeded; you're now discussing my attire instead of me."

There are quite a few confused "What the hell?" looks around the table, maybe a few muffled laughs.

After a fairly long pause, Dr. Ratched declares, "This is a very serious matter. I'm not certain you grasp that."

I retort, "Oh, I understand how significant it is. I'm dead serious, which is why I'm wearing serious clothes."

I'm starting to have some fun; I know where this is headed, and I'm going to lead it there. Lovely Wife sighs, as she knows where it's headed as well. I whisper to her to stay out of the fray and that Ellen, our esteemed psychiatrist friend, is coming this afternoon and can hopefully sidetrack Dr. Ratched's plans for me, which I presume center around continued incarceration. Hopefully not worse.

Dr. Ratched, with a determined demeanor, continues by bringing up my "complaint stunt."

"You filed repeated complaints about light being shone in your eyes and causing you to wake up. We had a box full of them. What was that about?"

I explain, "I may have taken that a bit too far—let's blame it on the medications. However, unbeknownst to me, it was my first night on 'watch,' and I couldn't understand why every fifteen minutes a flashlight was shown into my eyes."

I continue, "The next morning, when the doctor took my vitals and did my bloodwork, he asked how I slept. I wondered if he was joking—how the hell did he think I slept having a flashlight shone in my eyes every fifteen minutes? So, he entered into the record 'poor sleep.' Then, I asked him why they opened the door every fifteen minutes, and he said, 'To make sure you are safe.' At that point, I figured it out: They were checking to make sure I wasn't trying to harm myself, or worse. Ironically, by waking me up thirty-six times to check if I was okay, they were actually increasing the odds of that happening."

Dr. Ratched responds, "Why did you inquire about the dosage of your drugs and whether they were fat soluble or water soluble—and why did you insist on discussing that with a doctor on a Friday night?"

I answer, "That's simple. I wanted to know because if a drug is fat soluble, the concentration in the blood remains relatively stable over a twenty-four-hour period, so once a day is okay. However, if the drug is water soluble, the blood concentration peaks right after being administered and drops quickly thereafter. To even that out, the drug should be given at least twice a day."

She stated that she had, in fact, looked it up. "Valproate is fat soluble, and lorazepam is water soluble."

Did I just detect a hint of humanity there?

I then assert, "So we agree, I get lorazepam twice a day?"

"Why not?" she responds.

I follow up with, "A half dose twice a day."

She nods her head.

I continue, "I requested to see a doctor on Friday night because I thought it was important to get the titration right. The most critical period is when you first start taking a drug. As you know, each person reacts to drugs differently; that's why you take blood so often in the beginning. If blood concentrations increase too rapidly, that can pose a problem, and if they don't increase fast enough, that can also be a problem. Just like Goldilocks, you want to get it just right. I thought it might be good to talk to a doctor, but I was informed that doctors didn't work on weekends. Well, guess what? *Mental illness does not take weekends off.*"

She forges ahead, "You persistently exhibit delusions of grandeur. You claim to be the CEO of a multibillion-dollar company, featured in a Harvard Business School case study, ran with the bulls, climbed Mount Kilimanjaro, completed multiple marathons, and even that you have a ten-foot, sixteen-thousand-pound moai head in your backyard that will become your tombstone, among other things."

I retort, "Don't forget the main reason I'm here: The pressure of putting on one of the year's most anticipated art shows in New York City triggered my full-blown mania and psychosis. No one has recreated the famous *9 Evenings at the Armory* since its 1966 premier."

She counters, "No, I haven't heard that one."

I exclaim, "Well, it's either all true or all a lie. Care to wager a dollar? That's my usual amount."

Unfazed, she presses on. "Furthermore, you flagrantly violated nearly every rule here by throwing a party last night. It was the most outrageous spectacle of which I am aware. You continue to exhibit impulsive and excessive spending, quintessential mania. How can you possibly justify that?"

With a smile, I calmly respond, "First of all, it was a great party, even epic. More importantly, it was the most cost-efficient therapy this hospital or any mental institution has ever seen. For seventy-six bucks, I was able to get twenty-two of your patients to laugh, smile, talk to one another, even dance. EVERYONE danced to "YMCA"—it was the most beautiful spectacle, as you call it, I've ever seen, or, better yet, been a part of."

I'm on a roll. "When is the last time you saw any of your patients do any of those things? By my calculation, it costs one MILLION dollars to house twenty-two patients for a month here. My seventy-six dollars brought them hope and joy and a reason to live. You spend a million to medicate them, so they won't die. Most of your spending is on paperwork. So, who is suffering from impulsive spending, me or you?

"That is a rhetorical question," Lovely Wife adds with a smile.

"Enough," Dr. Ratched proclaims and throws her pen on the table. She delivers her preordained verdict: "You will benefit from at least one more week here as an inpatient. We will review you on a week-by-week basis."

I am disappointed but not surprised. I pulled out all the stops: wearing my power clothes, freshly shaven, hair looking good, smiling, trying not to ramble, as I am prone to do.

She continues, "From the copious notes your caregivers are taking, you are a rule breaker, and the rules are meant for everyone's well-being. Your delusions of grandeur and compulsive spending exhibit no signs of abating. You continue to exhibit symptoms of a severe manic episode, with psychosis."

I hear some of her colleagues whisper, "Maybe we need to adjust his treatment."

No doubt they are talking about the nuclear option: shock treatment.

My parting words: "Thank you for listening. However, I have one last question: What's the difference between my stay here and Charles Manson's solitary confinement at San Quentin? Manson gets to go outside for an hour a day. I don't."

Their stunned silence fills the room as Lovely Wife and I bid them . . . adieu. I am then escorted back to my cell, or rather, my room.

The entire kangaroo court takes less than half an hour. As I open the door, a large crowd is gathered, extending down the hallway to my room.

With a big smile I announce, "You've got me at least another week." This is met with a great cheer and a rhythmic chant of "ONE MORE WEEK." I'm pretty sure I see Jason in the back joining in.

Lovely Wife sarcastically says, "Nice job. See you tonight," and heads for the exit. She really isn't disappointed that I will be staying longer; she needs the rest. I receive high fives all the way back to my room.

In the room, it hits me—the patient is not the only one affected by mental illness. It really affects a village. It starts with your significant other, who bears the brunt, and then spreads out to other family members, friends, business associates, and caregivers.

Jonah comes in a few minutes later and beams, "You have just been voted captain of the ward, by unanimous consent," which is a fancy phrase for no one objecting. It makes me smile: captain of the ship of fools. Jonah interrupts my reverie to let me know that lunch is being served in five minutes and to get moving since there's already a line at the door.

As we round the corner, I see the line is ten deep. However, I see someone waving me up—it's Kerin, mouthing, "Come on." I wave her off, deciding I'll tell Jonah later that Captain doesn't want special treatment; the honor of commanding the ward is reward enough.

Lunch is uneventful, except for the occasional party animal who comes over to thank me for the great time. I tell them it was a team effort. I avoid using an expression I hate: "There is no 'I' in team." The imbeciles who use it don't realize there's a "me" in there. I return to my room and decide I need to recharge the proverbial depleted battery. I notice that, along with *Alice in Wonderland*, Lovely Wife has given me another "safe" book, *Call It Courage*, authored in 1940 by Armstrong Sperry. This was my favorite book when I was growing up.

It was my "go to" book whenever I needed to write a school book report. I made it to the ninth grade before I was called out for reviewing a picture book. I don't want to have to give a spoiler alert, so I will just say it is about a Polynesian boy who lives on an island and is afraid of the sea. It's a must read that won many prizes, including the prestigious Newbery Medal in 1941. In 1973, Disney turned it into a film. Scrimshaw's review on Amazon reads, "It is an amazing American novel." I forget—did I mention the cannibals?

At this point, it's worth mentioning that I actually have well-hidden street cred as a blue-blood preppie. Aunt Paulene handed me a stack of documents and books about a year before she passed away, asserting I was descended from Thomas Rogers, a surviving passenger on the *Mayflower*, which landed at Plymouth Rock in 1620.

Among the trove was an application for me to join the Mayflower Society. All I had to do was sign. Yet, the unsigned papers remain buried under my release form from my second hernia operation. Though I must confess, if Marilyn Monroe had been alive at the time, I might have signed, given she was a descendant of John Alden, another member of the *Mayflower* crew.

Jason interrupts my reverie. "It's three o'clock. You have a guest coming in an hour."

I find this odd, as that's not visiting time, and they're strict about that. Who the hell could it be? I've got to check on Ben again, so I head over to his room. The mystery guest will be revealed soon enough.

As I look in his room, I see him sitting on the edge of his bed, head slumped down.

"Hey, Ben. Want some company?" I call out.

He grunts something unintelligible and shuffles to the door. We end up sitting on adjacent chairs in the hallway again. I ask him how he is doing.

"Still feel confused and tired, which is weird. I'm never tired and can't remember things," he admits.

I'm not sure how to respond. The ECT thing seems surrealistic to me. Am I in a bad dream? Will I awaken and find that the wicked witch (ECT) was made up? I hope so.

Eventually, I inquire, "Do you remember that you had a treatment this morning?"

"A treatment for what?" he asks.

I try to explain, "You're in a hospital because you have been feeling sad lately, and they thought they could help you."

Ben questions, "So what did they do to me?"

"It's probably better if one of the doctors or nurses explains it to you," I suggest.

"Have you had any of these treatments?" Ben asks.

"No," I reply, thinking, *No fucking way.*

Ben says, "Thank you. You are nice to me and have my back. I want you to know that I have your back too. NO one is going to hurt you; I'll make sure of that."

Just like in *One Flew over the Cuckoo's Nest,* where Jack Nicholson had Chief Bromden, the immensely strong, 280-pound, six-foot, eight-inch half-breed to look after him, I now have my own Chief. I thank him and ask if I can call him Chief. He nods, maybe thinking that's his real name. I tell him to call me Captain.

It's time to go to the central hallway meeting area to meet my mystery guest, and I see—wait for it—I need one more—wait for it—Dr. Empathy, a.k.a. the Queen of Empathy, in all her regal splendor.

It went something like this, "I talked to your wife, who, by the way, is a really wonderful person."

Let me hit the pause button for a second. Everyone says that about her, which to me implies that I am not a wonderful person, maybe even an asshole.

"You are so lucky to have her."

Another pause . . . *Well, isn't she also lucky to have me?* I think, *Hell, yes.*

Dr. Empathy continues, "She filled me in on your meeting this morning, and I decided to have a chat with your doctor."

"Dr. Ratched?" I ask with a straight face.

Dr. Empathy retorts, "Let's just call her Dr. R.," then continues, "I asked her to review the salient points, and she started off by saying that it was bizarre that you wore the 'power outfit.' It just emphasized your delusions of being the CEO of a major company."

"And?" I ask.

"I told her that you ARE the CEO of a very successful company, that Harvard Business School had written a case study about you, and that I had dinner with you and the author of the case."

"And?" I prod.

"Dr. R. was a bit taken aback and said, 'He was disruptive and asked for a doctor to talk about his meds, on a weekend. He was really agitated that there wasn't one available.'"

Dr. Empathy goes on, "I then let her know that your wife shared your diagram with me concerning staffing and that I thought you had come up with a very clever solution—the rotating schedule."

"Nice!" I exclaim.

She goes on, "I suggested to her that perhaps someone should write a short article for *Psychiatry Today* on that topic. The title 'Mental Illness Does Not Take Weekends Off' was clever and to the point."

Hot dog! I'm really relishing this. (Cut me some slack. I need to amuse myself every once in a while.) "Keep going."

"Dr. R. had quite a rant about moai heads, marathons, Mount Kilimanjaro, and running with the bulls. Your mythical art show and extravagant spending on a party also got a mention. I countered by sharing that I've seen your sixteen-thousand-pound moai head, I know about your running achievements and your successful climb up Mount Kilimanjaro, which raised tens of thousands of dollars for innovative cancer research and was chronicled in a front-page story in one of the Boston newspapers. I also informed her that I'm planning on attending your art show and hinted there was even more to your story."

Dr. Empathy then looks at me and says, "That your accomplishments were not delusions of grandeur, and you have had some pretty impressive achievements despite and because of your neurological differences."

I have to smile at that one. "You mean that crazy can be a gift?"

"Something like that," she replies. "Oh, yeah. I didn't tell her that you can sometimes be a pain in the ass. I'm pretty sure she has that one figured out."

"And the party?" I inquire.

"She was really, really upset about that, asking, 'How was that not breaking almost every rule and indicative of excessive, impulsive spending?'"

I agreed that it was unorthodox. However, seventy-six dollars wasn't all that extravagant. Other patients have ordered delivery before, and that there was nothing technically wrong with holding a Bible group meeting—after all, you are an ordained minister. (This is true, but it's too long a story.) There was no prohibition against playing music as long as no one was annoyed by the volume. And since everyone on the ward was there, no one seemed to be annoyed. I did add that there were no deleterious effects on the patients, and it seemed that most were actually positively affected.

"The last issue was very serious. I asked her if it were true that patients are not allowed outside and that you had been kept inside for seven consecutive days. That would be particularly egregious since you are clinically claustrophobic."

"What was her response?"

"She wasn't aware of the claustrophobia and thought it was safer for the 'patients under special surveillance' to stay inside."

Dr. Empathy further relays her discussion with Dr. R. "'So is that common practice for someone who is physically capable of going outside? In mental institutions, where the risk of suicide is already high, the absence of outdoor time should be viewed as a potential trigger for self-harm.' Dr. R. responded, "Um, I need to look into that,' at which point I thanked her for her time and came over to see you."

"Thank you, Dr. Empathy."

She smiles. "And how does that make you feel?"

I laugh, recognizing the inside joke between us, and say, "Good one," and burst into my favorite James Brown song:

Whoa! I feel good, I knew that I would now I feel good, I knew that I would now

So good, so good, I got you

On her way out, she turns, laughing, and says, “See you on the outside.”

Back to my room, Jonah informs me that Kerin and Chief want to join us for dinner, and we have about thirty minutes until it is served. I’m exhausted and take a nap, only to wake up to Jonah dripping water in my ear.

Smiling, he says, “I know it’s the nuclear option, a term you like, but you were comatose, and nothing else was working.”

I decide I’m not that hungry but in desperate need of a caffeine boost, so I grab the two cups of high-test joe that Jonah has procured for me, along with the Nestlés, and head to the cafeteria.

Kerin and Chief are already seated at what has become our usual table. I take both coffees and place them in the twelve-hundred-watt microwave. To heat them to 150 degrees Fahrenheit will take about two minutes. Once the microwave *dings*, I dip my finger in, and the temperature is about right. I pour in the two packets of Nestlés and stir. Within seconds, I feel rejuvenated, focused, optimistic, and better than good to go. The best medicine they dispense here, and they don’t even realize it.

Kerin mentions that the party is the talk of the ward. “Everyone thought you would be in big, big trouble.”

I confess that I’m just in big trouble, and that I have a friend in a very high place who bailed me out. I reveal that I do want to get the hell out of here. “So, from now on, I will be pretending to go along with their shit, and with a lot of help from my friends, I’m hoping to be released in another week.”

Stepping out of the cafeteria, I’m greeted by an unexpected surprise: Two very good friends of mine are visiting. The wife, Jamaican royalty, the husband, one of the top healthcare lawyers in the country. They are holding a stuffed unicorn—I love unicorns, and I’ll tell the unicorn story in a moment. They indicate that Lovely Wife is keeping them up to date.

Predictably, they add, “And by the way, she is the nicest person,” and I’m “so lucky to have her, blah, blah, blah.” Ugh, I’m going to have to hire her PR person.

Jamaican royalty poses the empathetically correct open-ended question: "How's it going?"

I respond, with a bit of pride, "Great! I earned my way into the country's premier insane asylum, where the worst of the worst are corralled, and somehow, I've been deemed the craziest of them all. I'm hoping to be inducted into the insanity hall of fame, alongside James Taylor."

They respond, "We wouldn't have expected any less."

Top healthcare lawyer then reassures me about the "little issue" I had at the annual outing of the prestigious We Heal the World Foundation at Fenway Park recently. Incidentally, he also happens to be the chairman of the board of said foundation.

I have a vague memory of something happening, but I choose to simply say, "Thanks."

They spot someone else waiting, hand me the unicorn and explain it is self-explanatory, give me a forbidden hug, and . . . bid me adieu.

Now the unicorn story. Typically, a unicorn is described as mythical, rare, and highly valued. It is depicted as a white, horse-like creature with a single horn on its forehead. The really cool part is that they can be found anywhere as they inhabit the realm of the imagination.

On to the good stuff. The Urban Dictionary defines a unicorn as "a single female interested in meeting a couple, described as such due to the rarity of finding said female." Don't shoot the messenger; I'm just quoting verbatim.

I have a feeling that I have another connection to the unicorn, a vague memory, a fragment trying to surface from my drug-induced haze. Aha, now I see it; there is a seven-minute YouTube video titled "The Crazy Hot Matrix: A Man's Guide to Women," first released in 2014. It has been viewed by millions, including a handful of women—Lovely Wife being one. While I neither endorse nor agree with its content, if you haven't seen it, it's worth watching so you can judge for yourself whether it's educational or just blatantly sexist and offensive. I'm going to give a spoiler alert here because I'm about to reveal the plot, which is necessary to explain the unicorn reference.

Dana McLendon teaches the "A Man's Guide to Women" course. He is, allegedly, an instructor at the Tactical Response Group, an organization that imparts "the mindset, tactics, and skills to prevail in a violent confrontation" to students "regardless of age, gender, occupation or race." McLendon proposes that there are two important criteria that men should use to evaluate potential danger when prospecting for dates or mates: hotness and craziness.

He illustrates his theory with a graph, where the x-axis represents the "hot" scale, "with the traditional 0 to 10 range," and the y-axis reflects the crazy scale, "ranging from 4 to 10, because what woman is not at least a 4 crazy." The hot–crazy line slopes upward, indicating a positive relationship between hot and crazy. On average, the hotter, the crazier.

The most intriguing area of the graph is where the women are rated high for hot and low for crazy—this is the mystical land where the unicorns roam. Dana suggests, "If you find one, capture it alive and send it to us so we can study her and possibly replicate it."

The video also offers a corresponding graph for women evaluating men. It is disarmingly simple—if a guy is really hot, 8 or above, but not rich, this is the fun zone; experiment but do not marry. However, if you find a man who is rich, marry him immediately, regardless of hotness.

Just as my friends are departing, I see my business partner, Ernie, striding over. It's weird—I can never predict which visitor will show up until they actually show up.

Grinning, Ernie quips, "Have they electrocuted you yet?" He possesses a dark sense of humor—one he seems to reserve just for me.

I counter weakly with a remark about his last name, a moniker for a rigid male organ.

He continues, "I dropped off your sketch of *Newton's Balls* with Paul at the stainless-steel fabrication plant. The place is amazing. Paul's like the Larry Bird of stainless steel." Ernie loves sports analogies. He shares, "Paul is really excited and has produced some 3D computer-generated models of the cradle, and he's in constant touch with the ball-bearing guy in Florida, Zach. However, they are waiting for your final rendering before they can begin fabrication."

I tell Ernie, "Excellent job. Let them know that they're invited to the art event, contingent on setting the balls in motion."

With a final, "Onward, dork," his affectionate nickname for me, he turns to leave, but not before I respond with my respectful tag for him: "Pecker."

I see Lovely Wife hustling over. She looks like a woman on a mission. She is carrying another book for me. Please, once again, let it be Harry Potter. I have a first edition *Harry Potter and the Philosopher's Stone*, and it was not easy to acquire. It was initially published in the UK on June 26, 1997. A friend in London had given me a heads-up that it was getting a lot of buzz there and suggested I purchase a first edition since it could someday be worth a fortune. I did buy it, and it is worth a fortune.

Although I'm not surprised that the tome isn't a Harry Potter book, I am taken aback to see it is the Bible. Not just any Bible, but my family Bible dating back to the 1800s. Inside the cover is an inscription from my great-great-grandfather, Alanson Webster, dated 1857: Mathew 7:7, "Seek and you shall find." Fitting, since Lovely Wife had to search the attic long and hard to find it. I hadn't seen it since it was passed down to me over thirty years ago by my great-aunt.

With a smirk, Lovely Wife says, "Now that you're leading a Bible group, I thought this would come in handy."

She announces that she has to run, since our Bernese mountain dog has swallowed yet another sock and needs to be taken to Angel Memorial Hospital, Boston's finest. Of course. She has her priorities straight, but I hope we're not up against a repeat performance: a $4,000 bill!

I ask her to bring me another hat on her next visit, since I misplaced the last one.

With a nonchalant "Sure," she bids me . . . adieu.

I lug the Bible back to the room.

Jonah is already there and asks, "What's that?"

I reply, "Our family Bible."

He repeats, "No, what's that?" and points to a yellow sticky note protruding from between two pages. Lovely Wife loves to use sticky notes. This one reads, "Philippians 4:13."

I open to the marked page and read aloud, "I can endure all these things through the power of the one who gives me strength."

Jonah looks at me intrigued. “So, what does that mean?”
I answer, “It means that without Lovely Wife, I am lost.”
Exhaustion sets in. I tell Jonah, “I’m done. See you tomorrow.”
He responds, “Roger that.”

CHAPTER 10

TRIPPING WITH JENNIFER LAWRENCE

DAY 8: TUESDAY, AUGUST 6

When I wake up, I head to the bathroom and smile. I've got my routine down to less than five minutes. My efficiency-fanatic father would be proud.

As I'm leaving the bathroom, Jason informs me, "You have a meeting at eleven o'clock. Don't wear your power suit—you made your point with that."

Now this is interesting. I suppose it could go either way. Are they planning to escalate my case and go with the "nuclear option" (ECT) since I'm deemed irredeemable? Or did Ellen's intervention make a difference? After all, she is a TED Talk goddess with a worldwide reputation for being the Queen of Empathy. The "don't wear your power suit" suggestion makes me think there won't be a large crowd, but I'll find out in a few hours. In the meantime, I pick up my new book:

In the beginning God created the heaven and the earth. And the earth was without form, and void.
And darkness was upon the face of the deep.
And the Spirit of God moved upon the face of the waters.
And God said, "Let there be light and there was light." And God saw the light, that it was good.
And God divided the light from the darkness.
And God called the light Day,
and the darkness he called Night.

Genesis 1:1

Right from the outset, there it is: God created bipolars. The darkness of depression and the light of mania—two conditions as different as night and day.

Enough of the Bible study. It's time to discover a little more about my roommate, Jonah. We decide to skip breakfast and just talk for a while.

Knowing Jonah's interest in comics and anime, I decide to kick off with, "So what's your origin story?"

Jonah understands the reference. "So, you want to know how I got my superpowers?"

"Exactly," I confirm.

He shows his literary chops by asking, "You want the short story, novelette, novella, novel, or saga?"

I shoot back, "Since we only have a short time . . ."

He finishes with, "Okay, the short story."

He grew up in a rich, mostly Jewish suburb of Boston, in the only Irish family in the neighborhood. His father is a lawyer and his mother a psychologist. He has a twin sister—the yin to his yang—who possesses an abnormally high emotional IQ. She's very popular at school, highly engaging, and totally chill. They share a few traits: Both are very intelligent, and oddly, in Jonah's case, decent athletes.

During his junior year he became so proficient in digital art that in his senior year, he was offered a show at a Boston gallery. With the added stress of college applications, his schedule became so packed that he stretched his day by sleeping less and less and becoming more agitated and distracted. Sounds familiar.

Shortly after he was accepted, via early action, to one of the elite Boston-area colleges, his mother sat him down for a serious conversation.

"Jonah," she said, "we all love you. You're intelligent, kind, and talented. But this year has been somewhat overwhelming for you, and we think you might need professional assistance."

This led him to a psychiatrist at MorAss General, where he received a diagnosis of hypomania, or "low" mania.

Jonah was prescribed a medicine that didn't help. Then two more, which only succeeded in giving him unpleasant side effects, such as headaches and nausea and diarrhea. This brings us up to his high school graduation.

"Jonah," I ask, "by any chance, did you go to your prom?"

He surprises me with, "Sure, with my girlfriend."

Huzzah! Score one for Jonah.

Things got progressively worse for Jonah from there, and he stopped sleeping entirely. Exhausted, he hallucinated that he was the reincarnation of da Vinci. This earned him the metaphorical "Do Not Pass Go" Monopoly card and sent him directly to . . . MrClean. He missed his graduation, a particular shame since he was to receive both the computer science and art award.

After three weeks, he was discharged, and then required two additional weeks of outpatient treatment. He was released a couple of weeks before leaving for college. His parents wanted him to take a year off—what the fancy people, like Ernie, call a gap year—but he argued that having undergone treatment and starting on new medications, he felt better.

Just before he left for college, he was faced with one last tough situation. He and his girlfriend had decided that they would remain best friends but would no longer be "in a relationship," as social media terms it. So, off he went to college, single, but with the added burden of "breakup depression." (Yes, it's a real thing.) The stress of everything ended him back in the psychiatrist's office for round four of ineffective meds. Once again, he spiraled up, took a leave of absence, and reached full mania. He ended up as my roommate at MrClean, with a diagnosis of Bipolar I, with mania and a side order of psychosis, just like me.

Just then, Jason pops his head in and announces, “It’s showtime.”

He leads me to a small conference room, without a table, with a woman sitting in a chair facing an empty chair. She gestures for me to sit down and introduces herself as Dr. Bigshot. She informs me that she oversees patient care at MrClean. Dr. Empathy must have indeed pulled some strings.

At this point, I knew it could still go either way. They could lighten up on me, or there’s still some chance of the nuclear option. I like the Qur’an’s version of the “Day of Judgment” over the Christian version. The Qur’an states, “God sets up a scale. All deeds, good and bad, will be placed on either side, and if the scales are heavier with good deeds, the person achieves paradise; otherwise, hellfire.” I have a fighting chance with this one. Much like civil law, it is the preponderance of evidence that matters. In other words, if you are 51 percent good and 49 percent bad, you go to the good place.

However, Christianity sees things differently, and it’s much more complicated. You are absolved of all prior sins when you become a Christian, but if you commit sins afterward, you MUST confess those sins AND take Jesus as your Lord and Savior. John 1:9 states, “If we confess our sins, he [God] is faithful and just, and will forgive us our sins and purify us from all unrighteousness.” Then the killer, John 3:16: “For God so loved the world that he gave his one and only Son, that whoever believes in him shall not perish but have eternal life.”

This one is a little iffier for me, particularly the part about taking Jesus as my Lord and savior. As a mathematician, I admire Blaise Pascal’s work, as it led to the development of both the calculator and the modern computer. However, later in life, I came across his genius breakthrough in philosophy, “Pascal’s wager.”

He argues that a rational person should live as though God exists and seek to believe in God. If God does not actually exist, such a person will have only a finite loss (some pleasures, luxury, threesomes, etc.) whereas they stand to receive infinite gains (as represented by an eternity in heaven) and avoid the infinite loss (an eternity in hell) suffered by the infidels. I'm with Pascal, and so believing in God is a no-brainer. I'm also all for confessing my sins to "God." However, I don't buy the "Jesus Christ is my Lord and savior" part. So, I'm screwed if that is a deal-breaker.

Dr. Bigshot interrupts my theological musings. "We have reviewed your case, and it is a complicated one. On the one hand, you still appear agitated, have either ignored or bent the rules, and have exhibited animosity toward your doctor."

I'm waiting for the "on the other hand." I'm liking this; it looks like the Qur'an version of justice may be doled out.

"On the other hand, for a patient on serious medication, you are showing a high level of lucidity, observational skill, and insight. Some of your suggestions are quite good."

"I am revising your treatment to the following: You can have cellphone privileges, but you must follow the cellphone protocol. The camera will be disabled, and it must be placed in the charging station all night. You will be allowed to join the group that goes outside for an hour in the afternoon."

At this point I can't help but grin, ear to ear.

She goes on, "You can take art class for an hour a day, and you can go to the entertainment room."

The last one is a surprise, since I didn't realize there even was an entertainment room.

Dr. Bigshot then adds, "Conversely, you cannot order in food, disrespect your doctor, or disobey either the actual or spirit of the rules and regulations. If you agree, we will assess your case in one week, and I will make the final decision on whether you stay or go."

I figure I can work with that.

Since I am partial to one-word answers, I respond, "Agreed."

As I leave the conference room, I see Kerin and Jonah waiting.

Kerin, looking anxious, asks, "So?"

I relay the verdict, "Good for me, not so good for the ward. I get full privileges, but . . . no more parties."

They let out a collective "Noooooo!"

Jonah appreciates that it's great news for me, but they'd rather have me stay around longer.

Kerin looks at the clock and says, "Time for lunch."

On my way, I stop by the event board in the hallway and see a sign-up for the 1:30 p.m. outing. There's one slot left, and now that I'm allowed to sign up, I grab it.

I find it puzzling why they limit the outing to only ten inmates. If they acknowledge the therapeutic value of going outside and getting a little exercise, why restrict it to just ten?

With that logic, they should limit the meds to only the first ten who show up. Better yet, how about limiting ECT to just the first ten to sign up? Actually, they wouldn't have a problem with that one, since nobody would sign up.

Lunch goes by without incident. I decide to grab a couple of high-test coffees and Nestlé packets and take them back to my room. Caffeine really has been my secret weapon. My copious intake, probably close to a thousand milligrams a day now, has enabled me to partially offset the lethargy and fog brain induced by the meds. Another advantage, I realize, is that I haven't suffered any headaches, a common complaint on the ward. Over the years, I've often asked doctors why more research isn't conducted on coffee, given its significant and widespread benefits.

Their universal response: "Because no one will fund the research. It's a readily available, inexpensive commodity."

To which I respond, "Bullshit."

They need to look at things differently. There exists a substantial potential source of research funds, billions of dollars—actually, billions of Swiss francs. It comes from a company with a culture of high-quality research—and they would greatly benefit from the scientifically rigorous proof of the health benefits of coffee. They're already conducting in-house research to counter the negative narratives about coffee, such as "It causes cancer," "It's harmful to the heart," or "It's a diuretic," all of which have been debunked. And who might this potential benefactor be? Some of you septuagenarians might remember the jingle Farfel the dog sang in the 1956 commercial, "N-E-S-T-L-E-S, Nestle's is the very best."

That's right, Nestlé, the one that makes my cacao powder, is the company doctors should be courting. I have visited their headquarters in Vevey, Switzerland; it is like something out of a James Bond film. I was both shaken and stirred by the experience. Now, on to the data: Nestlé generates twenty-five billion dollars in coffee sales a year, which is a quarter of their total revenues. They make a profit of twenty cents on every dollar of coffee sales, which translates to five billion dollars in coffee profits. I estimate that they already invest half a billion in coffee R&D per year; they could do more. Research doctors should be beating a path to Vevey.

Speaking about beating a path, I rush over to the rendezvous point for my first venture into the outside world in eight days. I am really looking forward to the walkabout.

Apparently, you walk around the entire medical facility. I can't wait. It will serve as excellent reconnaissance for plan B—the great escape—if things go off the rails and I'm scheduled for shock therapy.

A male nurse, whom I don't recognize, lines everyone up in the sign-up order.

He looks at me and says, "You didn't sign up. You can't go."

Incredulous, I respond, "I did sign up. I was number ten."

He parries, "Your name is crossed off; number ten is Tommy." I consider arguing the point, but cave in for two reasons: a) it would conflict with my deal with Dr. Bigshot, and b) I'd likely lose the argument anyway, as I have no proof. It would be better that my enforcer, Chief, have a little "conversation" with Tommy later. Moreover, tomorrow I will hover around the bulletin board to make sure this doesn't happen again.

I then see Jason just shaking his head, saying, "I'll see you tomorrow on the outing."

Art class beckons. I enter the room and find the attendees haphazardly arranged around a large table. I'm relieved to see Kerin, who has decided to join the group as well, smiling and patting the seat next to her, which I promptly take.

The teacher greets us with, "Nice to see you. The materials are all on the table. Please be careful and respectful of the group."

I scan the room, and my eyes are glued to Elmer's. As any gluephile knows, Elmer's Glue was invented by the Borden Company in 1947. The brand name has an interesting backstory. Borden was primarily a dairy company, and their mascot was Elsie the Cow. After a decade, the marketing whiz kids at Borden decided to spice things up. Elsie would get married to . . . Elmer. The happy couple had two children, Beulah and Beauregard. Elmer's Glue is famous for being the safest—it's childproof and edible, a theory I test when the teacher isn't looking.

Next, I decide to create a rainbow. I love rainbows. A common misconception is that Sir Isaac Newton, of gravity fame, produced the first rainbow by passing light through a glass prism. However, someone beat him to it—Mother Nature. For a billion or so years, nature's own prism, a raindrop, has been creating rainbows. When the sun's rays pass through a raindrop, a seven-colored spectacle appears, invariably eliciting awe and delight. The viral video from 2010, with fifty million views and counting, featuring Paul "Bear" Vasquez's enthusiastic reaction to a double rainbow in Yosemite Valley, showcases this perfectly through his ecstatic cries of, "Oh my, oh wow, wow, wow, double rainbow, double rainbow across the sky," followed by, "It's a double rainbow, double rainbow. What does it mean?" He knows, it's just beautiful, more priceless than gold, and the definition of ecstasy—and we all want to have what he had.

I gather the necessary material for my rainbow: a sheet of letter-size paper, Elmer's Glue, rolls of crepe paper about an inch thick, and a black crayon. In my head, I can hear seventeen-year-old Judy Garland singing the iconic song "Over the Rainbow" from the *Wizard of Oz* movie. She was famous not only for singing this song, but also for her five marriages before her untimely death at age forty-seven. This one's for Judy.

Somewhere over the rainbow, skies are blue
And the dreams that you dare to dream, really do come true
Someday I'll wish upon a star
And wake up where the clouds are far behind me
Where troubles melt like lemon drops
Away above the chimney tops, that's where you'll find me

"Over the Rainbow," *The Wizard of Oz*, 1939

With the song echoing in my head, I begin crafting my rainbow, guided by my old friend, Roy G. Biv. Roy is the key to deciphering the colors of the rainbow, as well as their order: the acronym ROYGBIV, for red, orange, yellow, green, blue, indigo, and violet. Fortuitously, all seven colors of crepe paper are available on the table. But which color goes on top? A quick Google search, courtesy of my newly acquired phone privileges, reveals that red is on top, forming the outer edge of the semicircle that makes up a rainbow, making it the longest segment. To fit my rainbow on the eight-and-a-half-by-eleven-inch piece of letter-size paper, in landscape orientation, I opt for a diameter of ten inches. This means the red strip will be ten times half pi inches long, about sixteen inches.

Each successive rainbow-colored strip is about an inch shorter, given the decrease in the diameter of the arc. Although I could do a deeper dive into the math—something I actually enjoy—I'll stop here. Maybe I'm a little like Rain Man, played by Dustin Hoffman, a math savant on the spectrum.

There it is—the elephant in the room. Maybe I'm bipolar, with a side order of psychosis and a splash of autism. I glue the pieces in place, and a real rainbow emerges from the paper. The coup de grâce: In the open space beneath the violet semicircle, I use the black crayon to sketch two small eyes and a straight-line mouth—an expressionless, enigmatic face that doesn't clearly indicate happy or sad. A reflection of BP, perhaps? It's perfect, rivaling Leonardo's *Mona Lisa* "smile." I am amazed at how it all is working out—not only working out, but it is also a work of art.

The art teacher comments, "Nice job," and I strut triumphantly out of the room as she takes a few notes.

In the hallway, a new inmate approaches me, having heard about my skills in the investment business. She proclaims that she's a multibillionaire, attributing her fortune to being an early Bitcoin investor. For the record, I think Bitcoin is a total Ponzi scheme, but that's a different book. She proposes that I manage her assets. At first, it seems plausible—bipolar people may be crazy, but they are often very successful, and HUGE risk-takers. I say that I will consider it. However, a few minutes later, her story changes—she now credits her wealth to cracking the cold fusion puzzle, patenting it, and selling it to a consortium of electric utility companies for . . . ten billion dollars. Can you spell DELUSIONS OF GRANDEUR? Now I have an inkling of why my story might seem suspect.

Feeling drained after a long day, I make my way to the cafeteria to get . . . oh no, it's past 4:00 p.m. and too late for the caffeine kick I desperately need. I can't believe I overlooked the all-powerful joe, and I've got no reserves in my room. Dejected, I retreat to my room.

Jonah is on his bed, engrossed in a Japanese comic book, *Manga Sutra*.

As Jonah so succinctly puts it, "It's a 2008, 383-page, adult comic authored by Katsu Aki. It actually has a plot, centered around two twenty-five-year-old Japanese newlyweds, Makoto, the husband, and Yura, the wife. They have no experience with sex. It offers a blow-by-blow guide, complete with detailed visuals, to aid the couple.

I advise Jonah to ditch the book, since his ex-girlfriend will be visiting soon. I generously volunteer to take it off his hands.

He laughs and points to three cups of the high-octane stuff on my built-in shelf, my rocket fuel.

"Two for you, one for me," he declares.

I give him a thumbs-up, my highest expression of gratitude. I jog to the cafeteria, microwave the coffee, mix in the cocoa, stir, swallow my real medicine, jog back to the room, and get ready for dinner.

Jonah and I arrive early for dinner, wait for the door to open, grab our meal, and sit down at our regular table. Kerin arrives shortly thereafter, followed by a somber-looking Chief. They grab their dinners and join us. I recall why Chief is looking so grim: he's scheduled for his second "treatment" tomorrow. Curiously, the term ECT is never explicitly stated. Chief grumbles about how when he asked about the "treatment," he got a vague answer. Something like, "It will help you, feel better." Ben wonders if that is true, why does he feel so shitty? We wrap up dinner and head for our rooms to rest a little before our visitors arrive.

Visiting hour is like Forrest Gump's box of chocolates—you truly never know what you're going to get. I've always hated the chocolates with the gooey stuff inside. Does anyone like them? And, for some inexplicable reason, I loathe coconut. In walks my professor friend, Jay, who teaches my case study in his investment class.

He's the busiest person I know, juggling too many roles: teaching, mentoring PhD candidates, writing cases, consulting with several companies, hobnobbing with the power elite, advising the Fed, running mountain races, co-parenting two active kids, hosting cognac discussion groups with colleagues, and building his own outdoor sauna, all of which is just the tip of the proverbial iceberg.

Professor Jay is reassuring, as usual. He informs me that he's been here several times before—not as a patient, but visiting some of his students who had gone over the edge. We reminisce about some of the highlights of our shared history, including our race up Mount Washington and my "performance" during one of his teaching sessions of my case, which is still a topic of speculation among the faculty.

In his classes, he often invites the real-life "protagonist" of the case being studied—yes, they actually use that term—to sit incognito at the back of the classroom. This is easier than one might think, as other professors, who are considering using the case in their own class, often sit in as well.

There's one particular stunt I pulled during his class that's worth mentioning. It demonstrates my lack of respect for academic protocol, or pretty much any protocol for that matter. As the class discussion unfolded, some of the students began critiquing the central theme of the case, an investment product that I had conceived. In fact, a couple of "know-it-alls" may have called the whole idea BS, just marketing crap.

I do love the expression "know-it-all," first introduced in the early 1960s on the show *The Adventures of Rocky and Bullwinkle*. Rocky is a flying squirrel and Bullwinkle, a moose. In several of the episodes, Rocky would pause the narrative to introduce Bullwinkle, who would adopt the persona of Mr. Know-It-All to explain a phenomenon that had just occurred on the show, such as the physics of bird flight.

Bullwinkle's demeanor was arrogant and patronizing, as if explaining to a kindergartener. Okay, admittedly, some of my friends refer to me by this nickname. I embrace it and use it as one of my pseudonyms. When I start to "launch," I sometimes call myself Mr. Know-It-All.

After my professor friend finished presenting the case, he announced to the class that there was a special guest in the room: the protagonist of the case. I noticed several of the know-it-alls wince, realizing they had blown any chance of getting a job at my firm. As I began to walk onto the raised stage in March 2013, I was suddenly reminded of my crush de jour, Jennifer Lawrence. During the Academy Award presentations earlier in the year, Jean Dujardin had announced that Jennifer had won the Best Actress Oscar for *Silver Linings Playbook*, costarring heartthrob Bradley Cooper.

She wore an elegant white sleeveless gown, long and flowing, designed by Raf Simons for Christian Dior haute couture. She was a bit of a tomboy and not used to such couture. As she lifted her dress to climb the first of nine steps to receive her much-coveted, twenty-four-karat gold-plated Oscar trophy—wait for it—she fell face-first on the first step. At that moment, I realized the serendipitous brilliance of that fall. She was the sixty-ninth winner of the Best Actress Award—can anyone recall any of the other acceptance speeches?

For some reason, I wanted to be remembered by these students until their dying days, immortalized, part of their lore. So, what did I do? I fell face-first on the first step. There was a collective gasp; several students ran to help me. I thanked them, took the stage, and immediately shared my strategy for being indelibly etched into someone's memory. If a listener remembers even one thing from a presentation, you're doing better than 99 percent of all presenters. It worked for Jennifer Lawrence, and it had just worked for me.

A stunned silence followed; some were smiling, others shaking their heads. Once the class concluded and I descended the stairs, a crowd gathered around me. The only topic anyone wanted to discuss was the fall. Most agreed that it was a brilliant way to recover from an embarrassing stumble, demonstrating an uncanny ability to think on my feet at warp speed.

One student asked directly if I had actually planned the stunt. "You didn't really do that on purpose, did you? No one in their right mind would do that."

He was right about that.

As he gets ready to leave, Professor Jay casually mentions, "By the way, we're running the Sierre-Zinal Mountain Race next year in Switzerland. You have a year to train," and takes his leave.

Now that I have phone privileges, I Google the Sierre-Zinal Mountain Race. It takes place in the heart of the Swiss Alps, covering 31 kilometers (19.2 miles), with 2,200 meters (7,260 feet) of vertical gain, all for just ninety-five Swiss francs (a hundred bucks). I'm liking this. I've done a lot of similar things, but never in the Alps. The trail goes along mountain ridges and maybe even a glacier or two.

As he's about to go out the door, I shout, "Let's do it!"

He raises his fist and shouts, "Upward."

Just like a revolving door, my professor friend departs, and Lovely Wife appears.

She smiles and asks, "How did it go with Jay?"

"Great," I reply. "We're running a 31K race in the Alps next year. Want to come along?"

"I'll take a pass," she responds.

"I'm sure Barry will join you." I feel sure of it too. Barry is not one to miss a great adventure, even if it isn't on his bucket list. After all, it is bucket-list worthy. Warning, detour ahead. I really shouldn't go here. However, once again, if you want to understand how the mind of an unfiltered bipolar works, or rather, doesn't work, then you'll have to indulge me with the notion of being "bucket-list worthy."

As I've mentioned, the show *Seinfeld* was brilliant. Whether the genius behind it was Larry David or Jerry Seinfeld is a debate for another time. The show took the everyday mundane and elevated it to the exosphere. Most people would say "elevated into the stratosphere," which is only thirty miles high, while the exosphere is . . . six thousand miles high, significantly more impressive. Sorry, I just took a detour within a detour.

In one episode, Elaine, played by Julia Louis-Dreyfus, Jerry's on-again, off-again girlfriend, is running out of contraceptive sponges. For the prudes, a contraceptive sponge is used as a form of birth control. Elaine is prone to being promiscuous. Her dwindling supply of sponges forces her to become increasingly selective about her "dates." Those who make the cut and are deemed "sponge worthy" earn a notch on her Hermès belt.

Lovely Wife keeps it brief, explaining she has some work to do on the Marilyn Dress exhibit for the postponed show. Note to self: Talk to Barry about the Sierre-Zinal Mountain Race when he next visits. Lovely Wife hands me a book; I'll look at it later.

Back in the room, I notice the book *Empathy for Dummies* that Lovely Wife had given me. I pick it up and turn to the chapter on the Golden Rule: "Do unto others as you would have them do unto you." I then grab the Bible and find the citation, Matthew 7:12. My mind cycles back to shock therapy, with an intermediate stop at "invisible fence."

To keep dogs safe and contained within your property, companies sell a collar that delivers an electric shock if your dog tries to cross a wire buried around the perimeter of the dog-safe part of your property. Being a tech guy and wishing to prevent our first dog, a Rottweiler, from wandering off and possibly doing damage to a neighboring child or two, I ordered one. I also liked that the inventor of the "invisible fence," Richard Peck, a fellow Pennsylvanian, received the patent in 1973.

A dog learns not to get too close to this wire, as the resulting shock is, well, shocking. The voltage used to generate an electric charge potent enough to make a hundred-pound Rottweiler yelp in surprise is a mere three volts. I figured that if I was going to subject my dog to this, I should try it on me first. So, I fastened the electric collar around my neck, approached the boundary line, and . . . shrieked in pain. Not just a shriek, but my arm twitched involuntarily. The voltage used in ECT is . . . more than thirty times stronger. However, the human who receives ECT doesn't shriek as they are under anesthesia.

Perhaps the Golden Rule should apply in this case. Those who administer ECT to others should have ECT administered to them first. As Dr. Empathy, a.k.a. Ellen, suggests, doctors ought to exhibit greater empathy, defined as the ability to understand the feelings of others. It's hard to truly imagine something without experiencing it.

Just before bedtime, I concoct an ingenious enhancement to my plan B, my exit strategy, should it ever become necessary. I can hardly wait for art class tomorrow. If my rainbow elicited awe today, tomorrow's masterpiece will emote tears.

To Jonah, I say, "Until the morrow."

He responds, "I'll see you anon."

It's great to have an art and computer science major, with a minor in theatre, to appreciate my literary references.

CHAPTER 11

"MY DOG DIED | HE WAS MY BEST FRIEND"

DAY 9: WEDNESDAY, AUGUST 8

I'm up at 6:30 a.m. Jason escorts me to the bathroom. On my way out, I turn to leave, and Jason presents me with several cans of shaving cream.

"For the stash," he says.

I feel like I've won the Powerball. This is no ordinary shaving cream; it's a 1.5-ounce can of pure heaven. Small enough to take on an airplane, DawnMist Shave Cream promises "rich lather for a comfortable shave."

It's the best thing in this place, aside from the caffeinated coffee. It goes on smooth, is rich and thick, and stays that way. It soothes my soul even more than my face.

I need to find a secure hiding place for my stash of shaving cream. In here, they're as valuable as cigarettes in prison—the gold coin of the realm. There's no ideal place, so I take a gamble and hide them in my room, where after all, only authorized individuals are allowed. I learned that the hard way. If they're still there by the end of the day, I'll hand them off to Lovely Wife tonight.

Off to breakfast, where I concoct my special mocha and enjoy a plate of scrambled eggs with salt and pepper. I spot Chief, sitting alone, and go over to his table. He looks dejected.

"What's up?" I ask.

"ECT at eight. No breakfast for me; otherwise I'll throw it up," he says.

"Did they tell you the schedule?" I inquire.

He grunts and says, "Third one on Friday."

I interrupt, "I bet nothing on the weekend."

He goes on. "Yup, then Monday, Wednesday, and Friday of next week and I should be done."

I just hope he won't be done, done.

Chief confides that he dreads the pounding headaches, memory loss, and disorientation that come with the treatment.

He continues, "It sucks, but they say it will make me better? I trust you. Will it?"

My conundrum raises its ugly head again. I'm fully aware of the power of the placebo effect, and if ECT is effective at all, I believe it's most likely due to that. In response to the "billion-dollar question," I respond, "Yes." Because if a lie has the power to become the truth, can it still be considered a lie? I tell him we'll catch up later and have dinner with Kerin and Jonah.

I round up Kerin and Jonah and suggest we meet in the activity room for a movie.

We watch *Back to the Future*. A timeless classic, starring a pre–Parkinson's Michael J. Fox as Marty McFly and Christopher Lloyd as Dr. Emmett Brown. Despite the clever use of time travel, for me, the most impactful aspect of the movie is Christopher Lloyd's hair. Since its premiere in 1985, worldwide, particularly Japan, people point at me and say, "Isn't that the crazy scientist from *Back to the Future*?" It turns out Doc Brown, and I have exactly the same hair. I didn't take that as a compliment.

Afterward, we head to the bulletin board, and I'm the first to sign up for today's outing. To prevent any mischief, I decide to stick around. Once again, Kerin kindly offers to bring me a sandwich after her lunch.

When I ask them about joining the field trip, they consider it and decide, "We'll see how your experience goes, maybe tomorrow."

In a fairly regular stream, campers drift by to add their names to the list, staring at the new name, "Captain," at the top. I inform them, "I'm Captain, and I'm not happy that someone crossed my name off the list yesterday. That someone is named Tommy. If you are Tommy, keep on walking."

With a couple of minutes to go, all ten of us all line up according to the sign-up order, me at the front. Two nurses arrive with one minute to spare. Jason takes his position at the front of the group, and Nurse 2 takes up the rear, creating a "nut sandwich."

"Let's move, single file into the hallway," Jason commands.

He unlocks and opens the door. Following his lead, we enter a well-lit hallway about twenty-five feet long, with a door on each end. When everyone is in the hallway, Nurse 2 lets the door close with the usual *click.* Jason then unlocks the second door, and we follow him into a stairway, which spirals downward. Two stories down, we reach another door that Jason unlocks, leading to an underground hallway.

The hallway meanders with multiple forks; sometimes we take a left, sometimes a right. Finally, we enter a junior high school–sized gym through yet another random door. No way! That's totally surprising. The half-court basketball court is center stage, with several balls strewn about.

Jason yells out, "Ten minutes, and then we head outside!"

There's also a treadmill and a StairMaster against one wall. What an unexpected treat.

As I move toward the treadmill, Jason warns, "Don't bother. They're busted and haven't been fixed in over a year."

Baffled, I ask, "Why don't they fix them?"

He shrugs, replying, "I guess it's not a priority."

I respond, "You mean they just don't give a shit."

I drift over to the group "shooting" hoops. The quotation marks are because no one hits the rim or net or even gets within five feet of the basket. I was going to suggest we choose sides for a game using the playground pickup rules. But a pickup game would be a cruel joke given the circumstances.

After what feels like an eternity rather than ten minutes, Jason mercifully blows his whistle.

"Everyone, line up by the door and follow me out," he instructs, with Nurse 2 in the rear.

I stumble outside, and the sun is blinding. I imagine it must be what the thirty-three Chilean mine workers who were trapped underground in 2010 for sixty-nine days felt, except we don't get sunglasses.

But who cares? I am outside at last, outside at last, thank God almighty, outside at last. We self-select into one of two groups: Jason's group is for the fast walkers, so I nickname it the fast group; the other group is, well, the slow group. I join the fast group for various reasons: I am fast, but more importantly, I've always wanted to be part of the "fast" or popular crowd.

We set off on our adventure, walking in a counterclockwise direction around the haphazardly arranged buildings of the hospital complex, seemingly designed by a former patient. Squinting, I see the trees from a new perspective.

Leonardo da Vinci's fascinating rule about trees has aways interested me: the combined thickness of a tree's branches equals the thickness of the trunk they sprout from. He described trees as fractals, with the branches and even leaves forming repeating patterns at different scales.

In contrast, novelist Hermann Hesse rightly stated, "Trees are sanctuaries. Whoever knows how to speak to them, whoever knows how to listen to them, can learn the truth." Which leads me to my hope that "the truth will set me free," John 8:31–32, sooner rather than later.

Living up to our name, the fast group takes the lead. Looking back, I notice some members of the slow group meandering aimlessly, one actually walking in tight circles. Maybe it's a side effect of their meds, but I suspect nothing does it better than ECT, to paraphrase Carly Simon.

While we are indeed faster, there's little interaction within the group, with several people actually engaging in soliloquies, or stated less pretentiously, talking to themselves. So, I decide to stick closely to Jason. He continuously monitors the group, muttering something about "herding cats." Thanks to my amateur astronomer father, I can discern our direction as we navigate around the buildings.

At high noon, when the sun is directly to the south, your shadow points north. Since it is close enough to high noon—which is actually one o'clock during daylight saving time—I can figure out which way is north. However, I'm most interested in east, since that's the direction of my escape route. East is a ninety-degree right turn from due north.

As I survey all the roads leading into and out of the hospital complex, I realize there are no fences or walls surrounding it. This is a really good thing—no, a really, really good thing. I was half expecting to encounter razor ribbon, or an electrified fence. Come to think of it, an electrified fence would actually make sense. You could get one last jolt of "treatment" on the way out, free of charge.

We end up full circle, back to where we started. Not surprisingly, the slow group is still there; they are more like the stationary group. I feel fortunate that I got some exercise and didn't have to wait for them to catch up—one of the benefits of a circular route. I glance at my phone and note that we still have fifteen minutes to go.

I ask Jason, "What's next?"

He replies, "We just hang out here for ten minutes and then head back."

I survey the surroundings and notice a pleasant surprise I hadn't noticed before: a beautiful courtyard with flowers of all colors, shapes, and sizes, even the elusive bird-of-paradise. These flowers are a rarity in New England due to the harsh winters that require their annual replanting. I speculate that a group like the Central Park Conservancy must be behind it.

I figure that the annual outlay for keeping the grounds at MrClean in a "healthy" state is about one million bucks a year. Given the usual 5 percent annual payout from endowment funds, they probably need a twenty-million-dollar endowment to support the effort. Finally, something is being done right here. I give a big shoutout to those unseen donors making this happen.

Well, maybe not so invisible after all. There's probably a plaque somewhere in the building acknowledging them by name, but I'll let it slide.

Being outside in nature's splendor is the best therapy I've received here, except perhaps for the epic party and my rocket fuel mochas. When the whistle blows, signaling the end of our outing, we line up again and retrace our steps back to the ward. Although the outing was great, I feel a bit sad hearing the final clink of the ward door closing behind us. We all do the "zombie walk" back to our rooms. I'm learning how to fit in, or at least getting good at faking it. Fitting in is not something I particularly like, but I now have to fit in to get out.

I take a short rest, whip a magic mocha in the cafeteria, then head to arts and crafts. On the table, I spot a round paper plate, the kind with the ridges along the outer edge—perfect for today's project. I grab it, along with a black crayon. The label claims it's edible, but given its "Made in China" marking, I don't trust it. Had it been a Crayola, maybe. They are manufactured in Easton, Pennsylvania, home of Hilltop College and dozens of former brothels. Back in the roaring twenties, the town pretty much ignored Prohibition. Thanks to its strategic location between Philadelphia and New York City, it had no shortage of repeat customers, many of whom were ironically the same politicians who'd passed Prohibition to begin with.

After experimenting with several variations for my project, I settle on one I think should work. On the top half of the paper plate, I write in crayon, "My Dog Died." Next, I draw a horizontal dashed line across the center of the plate, with "He Was My Best Friend" on the bottom half. This should serve the purpose. Now, this begs the question, what is the PURPOSE? Should I ever be scheduled for ECT, they have to give me some warning. At which point I will go with plan B—the essence of which is:

1. Bring my hat, sign, and phone on the outing.
2. Look for the right moment to make my break and use the phone GPS to take me to downtown Boston.
3. Sit on a street corner and panhandle with my "My Dog Died | He Was My Best Friend" sign. Get one hundred dollars in "donations" and buy a ticket for a Peter Pan bus to the Poconos.
4. Go visit Bell and Harold and hang out for a while and snail mail Lovely Wife with my whereabouts. After all, maybe "they" would be tracking my phone.

You might be thinking, *That is crazy. Would he actually do it?* Hell, yes, 100 percent. Better yet, all my coconspirators would love the ultimate caper. One issue would be how to break it to Lovely Wife, but she would understand. She has told me several times that "no way" would she allow them to administer shock treatment on me.

However, as I explained to her, my voluntary admission, with my plethora of signatures, allows them to do whatever they think is in my interest. She completely disagrees with this assessment. ("You were crazy when you signed them. It won't hold up.") She may be correct, and she would be a formidable foe to Dr. Ratched. I'd enjoy seeing that fight. However, better to be safe than sorry.

The arts and crafts teacher makes her rounds and checks out everyone's project.

Most are just scribbles, or lines drawn randomly on paper; the best actually use more than one color.

However, she lingers over mine, puts her hand on my shoulder, and empathetically says, "I'm so sorry for your loss."

I thank her, even though my dog is very much alive and naughty.

She jots some notes, no doubt something like, "He is sad today." Nothing could be further from the truth.

Back to my room and then off to dinner. I'm definitely settling into the routine. Kerin, Jonah, Chief, and I sit together. Chief is groggy and a bit nauseous but enjoys our company. We decide to watch another movie tomorrow. I suggest *Chariots of Fire*, about English runner Harold Abrahams's pursuit of gold in the hundred-meter sprint at the 1924 Olympics in Paris. The film's score, composed by Vangelis, should appeal to Kerin's musical aesthetic, the beautiful English architecture should interest Jonah, and Ben would enjoy the high level of athletic competition. All are in agreement.

After dinner, I have my first visitor, Barry the lawyer. When asked how he's doing, he tells me he's keeping up his running and "misses our friendly competition." Sure he does, bullshit friendly. Twenty years ago, I could beat him easily, which he didn't like, since in high school he was a state-ranked forty-yard sprinter and a decent hundred-yard dasher.

So, yeah, I beat a pretty good runner, *every single time,* and it must have driven him crazy. I suspect his frustration might have led him to train secretly with a professional coach, just like Abrahams. His day came on Sunday, October 30, 2005, at the Halloween Hustle 5K in Newton, Massachusetts. Day turned to night for me, and night turned to day for him; he beat me every single race thereafter.

Recalling this, I reply to his "misses our friendly competition" comment with a smile and tell him I just might be going for a run soon. I tell him to "wait here" and return with my freshly made "My Dog Died | He Was My Best Friend" sign. He corrects me, noting that my dog is actually female. Wow, pretty good observation for a 153 IQ.

I quip, "This is Massachusetts; she self-identifies as a he." Also, I thought it would be creepy for a homeless man to have a female dog. He kind of figures out what I might be up to and suggests, with a wince, "Don't do anything stupid."

"Never," my response.

Barry leaves; Lovely Wife enters.

She begins with, "Before I forget, here's the hat." Then she updates me on the show, relaying that "Jack wants to know where the different exhibits will be set up in the first part of the show in Chelsea. He needs to know exactly how many separate elements there are, and how much space each one needs."

I tune out a bit and just hear "blah, blah, blah."

"Are you listening to me?" she asks with a touch of annoyance.

"Sorry, the drugs make me spacey," I offer, and get that "Sure, right" look in return.

I plead that I really need to see the space before I can figure all that out. She reassures me that Jack, having handled this sort of thing many times before, will take care of the logistics. She also offers to help, reminding me that she organized dozens of events during her tenure as the Smyth College Social Club of New York City Chair. In fact, I remember that well, since we met at one of those events. However, until just now, I hadn't realized there were dozens; I'd thought I was her one and only. I recall that Jack used to produce shows at Studio 54, and he mentioned having choreographed "some weird shit."

What the hell, let's see what they come up with. Studio 54 meets Smyth College. I return to my room, Jonah is fast asleep, and I decide to join him in Lalaland. And then . . .

CHAPTER 12

"DO NOT LEAVE OUR SON ALONE"

DAY 10: THURSDAY, AUGUST 9

A piercing fire alarm jolts Jonah and me awake. We bolt into the hall, where we're met by blinding, flashing strobe lights and a shrill, pulsing alarm that reduces what's left of our brains into mashed potatoes. My first thought is that it must be aliens preparing us for their next feast. We are no doubt a delicacy on Planet Moron, where the hospital management must have originated. Most everyone is staggering around and bumping into each other—I guess the "no touching" rule is waived for now. Instinctively, I sniff the air for the pungent odor of smoke because we know what's in the vicinity of smoke. But there's nada, only the usual stringent aroma of chlorine they use to keep the ward sanitary.

All twenty-two of us are corralled into a holding area, including those on death row. The pain is excruciating, and I beg, "Someone make it stop, please, please make it stop." Several of us assume the fetal position on the floor, while Slugger looks like she's having a seizure. Kerin, Jonah, and Chief gather around me, each looking terrified. Given my recent model citizenship, I politely approach the night nurse to pose a question; however, the blaring noise makes that futile. I resume my fetal position.

The fire alarm continues to flash and blast for twenty minutes—that's right, twenty fucking minutes. No one knows if it's "real or fake," but I'm leaning toward "fake" since there's still no evidence of fire. This feels like a form of torture, not unlike ECT but without the anesthesia. Finally, the nightmare ends, and we are led back to our rooms.

A couple hours later, a soothing voice announces, "Thank you for your cooperation. The alarm was part of a scheduled fire drill, a test of the system, and there's nothing to worry about."

Well, that's bullshit. There's no way you would schedule a fire alarm at 2:30 in the morning, particularly in an insane asylum. Moreover, the law mandates that, in a public building, only the fire department has the authority to deactivate the alarm once it has been triggered. I was the assistant fire warden at my company, so I know this shit. Once again, they are covering their increasingly fat asses.

This whole incident feels dubious—not being evacuated, making us stand directly beneath the deafening alarms, not telling us what the hell was going on, and keeping us in the dark for the entire twenty-minute ordeal. Several of us have issues with our hearing, and one inmate, Slugger, even had a seizure. The good news: She can probably skip her next ECT treatment. I have to get out of this place if it's the last thing I ever do, to paraphrase the Animals.

We gotta get out of this place If it's the last thing we ever do
Please move this to the next line.
'Cause, girl, there's a better life for me and you

"We Gotta Get Out of This Place," The Animals, 1965

Back to our rooms, and before I fall asleep, an important realization hits me: I can now rule out triggering the fire alarm as a possible escape. At exactly 6:30 a.m., I'm awake and escorted to the bathroom by Jason for my usual routine. The eerie silence from central command makes me a bit anxious; I haven't heard anything for a while. It could spell trouble, or perhaps it's a good sign. The fact that my vitals haven't been checked or bloodwork taken for three days must be a good sign too. Wouldn't they check if I were due to undergo general anesthesia?

At breakfast, I am the first of our group to arrive, securing our much-sought-after corner table. The corner table is usually the best one in any cafeteria or restaurant. What makes it so appealing? For starters, you don't have the riffraff pass by when going to or from their tables, and you are far from the boisterous drunks at the bar. Worse yet, some might be using the bathroom—not an appetizing thought.

The main advantage is that you have a full view of the room, and most importantly, no one can sneak up on you. If you happen to be a member of a crime family, this is literally a matter of life or death. "Crazy" Joe Gallo either didn't know this, or thought he was above needing it. On April 7, 1972, he was celebrating his forty-third birthday with his family at Umberto's Clam House at 129 Mulberry Street in New York City's Little Italy. He was seated at a central table, facing sideways to the door, and, thus, did not observe two well-dressed gentlemen as they entered, aimed their guns, and shot him several times. Gallo stood up, staggered outside onto the sidewalk, where he fell to his knees and then onto his face, and bled out. He died right there.

To this day, perky guides recount the story to tourists. They take a picture of each member of their group standing on the exact spot; I was one such tourist. The best quote I've found about the incident is, "If youse want good clams, youse goes to Vincent's down the street. He deserved what he got for havin' no taste." Had the Darwin Awards existed back then, he would have won, face down.

Why wasn't it obvious that someone might have wanted to kill Crazy Joe Gallo? After all, he did murder Albert Anastasia, the head of the Gambino family, and allegedly attempted to assassinate his own boss, Joseph Colombo, who was the inspiration for the Godfather. The verdict is out:

He had it comin'
He had it comin'
He only had himself to blame
If you'd have been there
If you'd have seen it
I betcha you would have done the same

"Cell Block Tango," ***Chicago*****, 1975**

After breakfast, we decide to reconvene in the activity room for another film. On the way back to my room, I line up for my daily medication, swallowing each pill in view of the nurse to confirm that I've taken it.

When I'm finished, as I turn to leave, the kind nurse reminds me, "Don't forget your afternoon pill. You're the only one who gets that 'special' treatment." Score one for me.

I choose *Ferris Bueller's Day Off*, a classic from 1986, as our group's film. Matthew Broderick is perfect for the role, and his closing lines are profound: "Life moves pretty fast. If you don't stop and look around once in a while, you could miss it." Others have stated it differently: "Stop and smell the roses," "It's not the destination; it's the journey," and the Zen philosophy "Living in the moment." I'll also throw in "Can't see the forest for the trees."

Upon reflecting on this, I realize that perhaps I've been missing the bigger picture. The big reveal is the answer to the question, "Why am I here?" I've been focusing too much on escaping rather than concentrating on the here and now. Perhaps I'm here for a purpose. The word *purpose* hangs in the air for a moment. *Purpose, purpose, purpose*—the word keeps echoing in my head, like the wheels of a slot machine spinning round and round. Finally, the wheels all come to a stop, and . . . jackpot. I now realize my purpose.

My search for a Homeric purpose began on July 8, 2005. On that day, I stood among three thousand participants, waiting for the mallet to strike the gong. Suddenly, thunderous, rhythmic shouts of BANZAI, BANZAI, BANZAI reverberated through the air. Startled, I looked to my left and saw my son, and to my right, Barry—yes, that Barry—and his two sons. We were the only gaijin in the crowd. We were standing at the starting line of the thirty-fifth running of the Mount Fuji ascent. A grueling thirteen-mile "run" with more than ten thousand feet of increasingly steep incline, covered with volcanic ash, which is like quicksand.

Mount Fuji is closed for one day a year to allow runners to ascend from the very bottom. There are ten stations along the way: the first station, at the bottom, and the tenth station at the summit. Standing at 12,388 feet, Fuji is the highest point in Japan and therefore closest to the gods.

As such, it is considered the most sacred place in Japan. Many Japanese attempt the standard climb, which takes several days. For those who reach the top, it is considered the spiritual pinnacle of their life, much like Muslims view circling the Kaaba in Mecca.

I found myself getting into the spirit of the moment, echoing the chants of BANZAI with a few of my own. I reflected on previous discussions with Barry about why we do these "stupid" undertakings. The answer now seemed apparent. You must embark on experiences that promote self-discovery. Without that, you will never really know who you are. Every journey to self-discovery begins with a single step. We were at the starting line of another epic journey; time to be enlightened by the Zen of the mountain.

The giant gong was struck, and with the air reverberating with its sound, we were off. Even though we were experiencing the "Zen" of the moment, the stations were actually Shinto shrines. We breezed past the first four stations, as this part of the race didn't involve much elevation gain—nerds might refer to it as the flatter part of Fuji's parabolic shape.

Chaos greeted us at the fifth station, the halfway point. A road circles Fuji at this level and provides vehicle access from all the surrounding towns. This was the designated rendezvous point with our families. I scanned the scene and spotted Lovely Wife sitting on the ground, clutching her ankle in pain. She shot me a glare that screamed, "It's all your fault!" with an implicit "asshole." Truth be told, it was my fault. She'd hurried to reach me from the bus drop-off spot a mile away and had fallen and badly twisted her ankle. Despite her pain, she hobbled to the meeting place to greet me. For the record, I have been reminded of this misstep dozens of times ever since.

We fueled up, but the fuel was a bit weird. For hydration, they handed us Pocari Sweat, a Gatorade-like drink that tasted as described. Bananas were stacked in meticulous piles, with trash cans designated for the peels. Etiquette in Japan dictates that you don't walk and eat at the same time, so everyone stopped to refuel. Intriguingly, a short distance on, they handed out chopsticks coated with rock salt. Trusting they knew what they were doing, I took two, started licking, and we kept on ticking.

From there, the race turned out to be much, much more challenging than we'd expected. The footing was treacherous, and with none of the signs in English, we simply followed the queue of other climbers that had formed. The incline was so steep that running wasn't an option; you could only manage to put one foot in front of the other. Metal cables were provided on the steepest slopes, which allowed us to pull ourselves up. Many competitors gave up. However, descending was even more dangerous than climbing, so they just sat there until either help arrived—or, worst case, they died.

As we scrambled over a ridge, we spotted a sign in English reading "Top," which sparked wild celebration. However, after a few seconds, confusion, then anguish set in—the sign also read "Eighth Station" in English. It was apparent there had been a translation error; we weren't at the "top" but actually had two more stations to go, the steepest of them all. To make matters worse, the mountain trail to the actual summit had been closed due to the race's time limit of four hours being exceeded. The officials explained, in Japanese, that continuing would have been too dangerous (*abunai*—I actually knew that word) to continue as it would have been dark before we could have descended the mountain.

Not one to be a rule follower, I committed an unforgivable sin and decided to go for it anyway. I left my son behind. I would later try to blame my poor decision-making on the altitude, dehydration, and exhaustion, which had combined into a state of delirium. Maybe Barry was to blame; after all, he hadn't tried to stop me. I was confident that, if necessary, I could present a borderline plausible insanity defense in court.

However, my defense would fall apart in the court of marriage. Lovely Wife had repeatedly warned me, "DO NOT LEAVE OUR SON ALONE." On a technical note, I would like to point out that my son was not entirely abandoned; he was with friends, initially Barry's two sons and eventually Barry himself. But, as the saying goes, that was a distinction without a difference. I was sentenced to yet another lifetime of shame and guilt.

Guards had been positioned to prevent race participants from circumventing the barricade they'd set up to prevent runners from continuing to the summit. Betting that they would allow non-racers to proceed, I removed my running number and casually sauntered past the guards, even giving them a nod. Astonishingly, they let me through. Onward to the top, the real top this time.

Upon reaching the summit, I found myself utterly alone—zilch, nada, daremo inai! It appeared I was the only one who hadn't gotten the email. Was I about to become a snack for Godzilla? Or was there a human sacrifice to the gods in the works? Or perhaps, was I simply the stupidest human on the mountain?

Who knew? Who cared? I had made it. But now, with mission accomplished, I had to get down in a hurry. I recalled the wise words of my mountain guide on Mount Rainier: "The getting up part is optional; the getting down part is mandatory. Most people die on the way down." My response to that was, yet again, "Onward," or more appropriately, "Downward."

There remained a possibility that I would salvage the situation if I could catch up with my son before he reached Lovely Wife at the fifth station. He would have to walk down slowly, which would take some time. After quickly doing the math, I figured that if I ran down, I might have a shot. However, a minor problem arose: Multiple trails led down, but all the signs were in Japanese—kanji, to be precise, which is impossible for a gaijin to decipher. 愚かな外人, for a relevant example, which translates to "foolish foreigner."

Unable to determine which path to take, I randomly selected one, leaned back, and started to sprint down the extremely steep slope, covered in meters-deep volcanic ash, known as scree. I had learned this lean-back technique on Mount Kilimanjaro, and I sincerely hoped I had learned it well enough.

I was flying downslope, leaning way back, and for a moment, I believed my plan might actually work—I was covering ground fast, really fast. However, I leaned back a tad too much, and then overcompensated by leaning too far forward, when . . . I tripped and launched into a forward roll, head over heels, down the slope.

Not just any somersault, but the mother of all somersaults. The slope, steeper than forty-five degrees—closer to sixty—caused me to accelerate rapidly down the mountain in a tight ball. Astonishingly, I managed to have a lucid conversation with myself as I tumbled down. Initially, I contemplated slowing my descent by stretching out my arms, but quickly realized that it would most likely have only broken both of them.

So, what to do? I concluded that I was going to die, and die spectacularly—perhaps even earning the coveted Darwin Award, a kick-the-bucket-list item. With no other real choice, I just went with it. As I gained speed, my body began to bounce from one roll to the next, like a ball cascading down a flight of stairs, each bounce higher than the last. My peaceful contemplation of my imminent demise was abruptly disrupted when I collided with a very solid object. I rolled sideways a few times before coming to a stop, on my side, curled up. As the adage goes, "Life comes full circle; you exit the world the way you entered"—in the fetal position.

Miraculously, I never lost consciousness and was still alive to hopefully tell the story. I opened my eyes and saw my right hand in front of me. I decided to try to wiggle the tip of my pinky finger, just to see the extent of the damage. But nothing moved. My pinky didn't move, my hand didn't move, my arm didn't move—nothing moved. That was not good news. I always carried a backup for these crazy adventures, which consisted of a fanny pack filled with a large sum of money, three credit cards, medical insurance card, contact information, bandages, ID, hotel information, and my phone.

The catch was, I was totally paralyzed. Hence, my phone, just inches away, was dead to me. After an extended period of time, I checked again—still paralyzed. Was this the way I was going to die? Having a nice, introspective conversation with myself? Interestingly, my life wasn't flashing before my eyes, contrary to the cliché. I had lived a full life, done some pretty cool things, had a great wife and children—they'd survive without me. I had checked off most of the items on my bucket list—and the imminent Darwin Award would be the cherry on top.

But wait, they would still be really ticked off about me dying in such a foolish, albeit epic, manner. So, I decided to strike one last deal. This was the conversation I held with myself, verbatim: "Okay, I know we haven't spoken before, but I'm certain you know me. So, here's the deal—I want to keep on going for a while. If you are the devil, you can claim my soul, but at least I'll have some real fun along the way. If you're the good one, then I'll commit to doing something that will benefit humankind—something big, really big. Either way, as a sign, let me wiggle the tip of my pinky." It occurred to me that this might be a pinky swear.

I waited a moment, then a little longer, and just an itsy-bitsy bit longer. I tried to move the tip of my pinky, and . . . it worked. Next, the whole finger—yes, it also responded. After a little while longer, I tested my hand and then my entire arm. YES! I decided to really push my luck. I attempted to move the pinky on my other hand, then the entire hand, then the whole arm. Yes, I was going to live—my cellphone was within reach. But where the hell was I? How would I communicate my location to someone? I only had the hotel's number, which wasn't particularly helpful. I had to motor on. I sat myself up, leaned on the volcanic rock that had halted my fall, got up on one leg . . . then fell down.

After a couple of iterations, I managed to stand, leaning on my new best friend—Rock. I took inventory of the damage. Miraculously, nothing appeared to be broken, although every part of me ached. My clothes were torn to shreds, and my body was covered with shallow cuts, etched by the volcanic rock that had broken my fall. Hardly any of the surface area of my body was spared. Why wasn't I bleeding out? Two reasons: The cuts were not deep, and the black volcanic ash, the scree, had cauterized the bleeding.

I wasn't sure which direction to head, but it didn't really matter; I just needed to go down.

Eventually, I would hit the road that circled Fuji at the fifth station. It turned out there were multiple fifth stations on the circle road. I had made it down to a fifth station, but not the fifth station I had first encountered. I must have looked like the only survivor of a cataclysmic blast. I walked gingerly up to a guardhouse that happened to be located there, where a young man, dressed in a uniform similar to that of our National Park Rangers, was stationed.

Without looking up, he pulled out a loose-leaf binder—a translation guide, with both Japanese and English versions of different questions.

The first question he pointed to was, "Are you lost?"

I gave him a thumbs-up.

The second was, "Are you a member of the military?"

I shook my head and said "Ie," which means "no" in Japanese.

Third, "Do you need help?"

"Hai," I responded, meaning yes. I then handed him my cell, wrote down my name, and gave him the business card of my hotel. He dialed the number and had a rather long conversation, of which I understood nothing except an occasional "hai."

He showed me our location on a map and pointed to where the hotel was. He finished with a "sayonara" and handed back my phone. Unfortunately, I was on the exact opposite side of the mountain from where I should have been. There were no direct roads leading to the hotel. It appeared to be at least fifty miles away. Ironically, as I later learned, I was right at the edge of Aokigahara Forest, also known as the Sea of Trees, the haunting home to the ghosts of the dead. This was the place where many despondent Japanese chose to end their lives by hanging themselves from the trees, with their dead bodies swaying in the breeze. Just the year before, a record was set—more than 105 bodies were found hanging, breaking the previous record of 78.

What the hell was I going to do? It was getting late, but just then I spotted my savior—a green and yellow taxi. This was good, really good. I walked over to talk to the driver; he took one look at me and frantically rolled up the window. I noticed the nice white doilies on the back seat and realized there was no way he was going to let me mess them up. I knocked on the window, and he waved his hands with a barrage of "Ies." I put my hotel card up against the window, but he still dismissively waved me away.

Finding myself without any good options, I decided to go with the "money talks" route. I was carrying money, a lot of it. I took out a ten thousand yen note, worth about a hundred dollars, and put it up to the window. He glanced at it and then launched another round of "Ies." I took out a second ten thousand yen note, and his gaze lingered longer, and . . . he unlocked the door and gestured for me to sit in the back. Before I'd even touched the seat, it was covered with black volcanic ash.

After about an hour of driving, I decided to call the hotel, and somehow managed to get Lovely Wife.

Her words rang through the phone. "I can't believe you left our son alone. That's unforgivable. I don't want to hear a single word from you. We have delayed dinner. When you arrive, dress in your yukata and be in the dining room by 8:30 p.m. The hotel has already informed me that you are alive, for now."

Her reaction was better than I had anticipated.

Back at the hotel, I made my way past the doorman, who backed away with a shocked look on his face, and headed for our room. I stepped into the shower, turned on the water, and noticed the shower floor covered with a red liquid. Then it made sense—when the volcanic ash that had been cauterizing my wounds washed away, the bleeding resumed. Fortunately, the cuts were superficial, and the bleeding soon subsided. I then donned my yukata, slid into my slippers, and joined Barry and our families for dinner. If Lovely Wife ever reads this book, it will be the first time she's heard "the rest of the story."

I have lunch with the usual suspects: Kerin, Jonah, and Chief, who is feeling good: no ECT today, one tomorrow, then it's the weekend, and the zapper gets weekends off. I wonder how many of my fellow campers are receiving the treatment. My guess is about one out of three. I Google the question "How many patients receive ECT each year?" and get one hundred thousand as the answer—and rising.

Jonah surprises me by announcing, "We are all going on the outing today."

Chief and Kerin had signed us up earlier. The three of them haven't ventured out since they got here, afraid to leave the "safety" of the ward. However, today, we are going as a group.

We return to our rooms and get ready for the great outdoors. Chief, Jonah, and I show up early at the bulletin board and wait for the nurses to show up. They arrive at promptly at 1:29 p.m., one minute before departure time. Jason is there; does he ever get a day off? Nurse 2 is also present.

Now that I am trying to fit in better, I politely ask Nurse 2 for his name.

"Tim," he responds.

He is quite a large guy, but I refrain from the ironic "Tiny Tim" moniker. But where is Kerin? She has only one minute until she gets locked in. At the last second, she rounds the corner with a big smile, looking every bit the diva she is.

Somehow, she has managed to apply makeup, and her hair looks, well, divaesque.

We walk through the labyrinthine tunnels below the complex and enter the gym for our ten minutes of basketball shame. Kerin suggests we have a little five-on-five basketball game. It's the four of us plus Joey, a new kid, who wants to join us, against the rest. We play by a modified rule: first to eleven wins, since the usual twenty-one will never happen. The game ends after five minutes, eleven to nothing. As it turns out, both Chief and Kerin played varsity basketball in high school.

Chief could have gotten a college basketball scholarship, but he was better at wrestling, and their seasons overlapped. The game is a thing of beauty. Jonah, Joey, and I never touch the ball. When our team has possession, Kerin passes to Chief for a layup, then Chief reciprocates by passing the ball to Kerin for a jump shot—*swish, swish, swish*. They never miss. On defense, they either take the ball away or block it if our opponents manage to shoot. The nurses watch in awe, not taking any notes this time.

After ten minutes, Jason blows the whistle. We line up, the door opens, and we step out into the sunshine. Alongside caffeine, sunshine has to be the best mood lifter. As the Beatles sang, "Here comes the sun, and I say, 'It's all right.'" Joey joins Kerin, Jonah, Chief, and me, and we head over to Jason. Today, we're not just the core of the fast group; we *are* the fast group. Since we don't know much about Joey, we encourage him to share his story.

He begins by thanking us. He's never been very successful in team sports, and he reveals that the basketball game was his first real victory. As an only child, Joey lives with his family in a large house on five acres in Lincoln, Massachusetts. That's where the old money hides.

His dad, a senior partner at a national law firm's Boston office, represents private equity and venture capital firms, while his mom is an editor of a prestigious medical journal based in Waltham, Massachusetts. Joey shares that he was diagnosed with attention deficit hyperactivity disorder (ADHD) at a young age and subsequently prescribed medication. Additional diagnoses of anxiety and Asperger's syndrome followed. His parents found that the only thing that would hold his attention for any period of time was playing video games.

Over time, Joey became somewhat of a legend playing League of Legends. His summoner name, the alias players use in the game, was Omega—the last letter in the Greek alphabet—chosen to suggest he would have the final word in the game. League of Legends is a five-on-five, two-team game, where each team aims to destroy the other team's headquarters, called a nexus, which is guarded by minions.

Joey's social interactions were almost exclusively with his team members, who he knew only through their anthropomorphic avatars in the game. He revealed that you can learn a lot about a person through their gameplay—at least the important stuff.

I ask, "So how did you end up here?"

Joey replies, "Well, our team was doing great earlier this year. I was going to attend Cal Tech in three months and figured it was my best shot at making it to the League of Legends World Championships before college could interfere. We were practicing twenty hours a day, seven days a week. I began feeling I actually was my character. The next thing I knew, I was here."

Sounds like a touch of mania with psychosis should be added to his diagnosis, but what do I know?

"Welcome to Summer Camp, Joey," I add.

The rest of the walk continues in silence, appreciating the sun, the breeze, the scent of the leaves, the chorus of birds. This makes you feel like life is indeed worth living. This is natural medicine that has been curing the blues since the beginning of time. It is an example of why I believe the mental health community has it backward. Once again, I'll get on my soapbox—a word derived from speakers who got up on an actual soapbox in Hyde Park, London, to pontificate on their pet issue. Instead of devoting their resources to preventing patients from taking their own lives, they should be providing them with reasons to live. Experiencing the wonders of nature ranks high on that list. Why was I denied this? Was it because I was a pain in their ass? Was it my ignoring their authority? Was it spite? Who knows, but shame on them.

We return to the ward on a natural high. Our group has grown to five. Five is a good number—we have five fingers and five toes, starfish have five arms, the chemical boron's atomic number is five, and humans possess five senses. Aristotle was the first to document the "big five," and listed them in this order: sight, hearing, touch, taste, and smell. Speaking of taste and smell, it's a reminder for me to drop by the cafeteria and grab a couple of cups of caffeinated coffee and a few of packs of Nestlé cocoa for my late afternoon and evening mochas before the 4:00 p.m. caffeine cutoff.

This gets me thinking: *Exactly how much caffeine am I consuming each day?* Earlier, I had observed the cafeteria staff put two heaping cups of ground coffee into a percolator that brews about twenty cups of eight-ounce coffee. Two heaping cups of ground coffee weigh about 200 grams. So, each cup contains 10 grams of coffee grounds, and given that coffee is 1 percent caffeine, that equals 0.1 grams or 100 milligrams of caffeine per cup.

Now, let's not forget the caffeine in cocoa, which manufacturers try to downplay—approximately 40 milligrams. Therefore, each of my mochas has about 140 milligrams of caffeine, and consuming six a day equates to 840 milligrams. Is that excessive? Not really; even children in Scandinavia consume a similar amount. The FDA suggests 400 milligrams is safe, but concedes that's just a guess, so 840 milligrams sounds about right for an overachiever like me. It takes fifty to a hundred cups of coffee before it is fatal.

Back in my room, lying in bed resting, I realize I am experiencing a sense of peace for the first time since I've been here. I'm no longer preoccupied with my great escape—though I'm certain it would have been epic, and the inspiration for a blockbuster movie titled *Escaping Insanity*, or something along those lines. Now, my focus is on supporting my fellow campers and preparing for my art show, scheduled in six weeks. GB, the gallerist, and Jack, the gallery manager, have been heavily promoting the event. The art critics are anxious to see what all the buzz is about. But there's still much to be done.

At this point, the "buzz" feels more like bees swarming around a honeyless hive. Will we all get stung by a madman's delusions of grandeur? Maybe, maybe not. I'm not worried—well, a tad worried, but I have a world-class team who can move mountains, or at least sizable mole hills. I realize how lucky I am. They can strip me of my clothes, take away my rights and my dignity, but the bastards can't rob me of my sense of humor—sophomoric as it may be, and however much it might annoy Lovely Wife. Yet, my best path to freedom is to be average, as hard as that might be.

Movie afternoon has caught on, with over half of the ward attending. I was considering having Lovely Wife sneak in some microwave popcorn, but then decided it might appear too partylike. I've also decided to let the rest of our group choose the movies from now on. Our group needs a name commensurate with our status. I've spent a lot of time in Japan, and like their term for a gang of five—they call it a *sentai*, which translates to "five-person task force."

Indeed, we are a task force, our mission being to get out of here in one piece, or perhaps two. Why two? Well, I came in here bipolar and plan to leave bipolar, and bi means two.

Kerin agrees to take on the movie selection role, knowing that I plan to leave halfway through the movie. I need to focus on the art show, but I can't withdraw from all activities, as it might draw the attention of management. Maybe if I lie low, take my meds without complaint, adhere to my morning bathroom routine, show up at all meals, and participate in the daily outing and other activities, I just might fly under the radar.

I head for the arts and crafts room; this may be my last class since I don't really like it or feel the need to make anything else. Lacking any great ideas, and since the rainbow was a big hit with the teacher, this time I'll do a simple sketch. It's two stick figures in a tug-of-war. Obviously, it's an analogy for the constant struggle of a bipolar man to keep a balance between the pull of mania and depression. Although not the masterpiece of my rainbow, it's good enough to get me a pass for the class. On my way out, I spot a stack of black marbled composition books, the ones we used in junior high. I ask if I can take one for sketching.

The teacher responds, "Of course. Also take a couple of crayons."

Done and done. It will be perfect for working on my project.

I head back to the room and get ready for dinner, which is fun as we relive the basketball game that will become part of MrClean lore. Jason, the friendly nurse, will make sure of that. We agree to split up Chief and Kerin for the next game to keep it fair.

Chief is nervous about tomorrow; it's Friday, and he has his third ECT treatment.

He asks, "When do you think they're going to let you out?"

Good question. This is day ten. I hope to get out after my second week, so, "Four more days," I respond.

He looks sad. "I think I'm in for at least two more weeks, maybe more."

Kerin nods, saying, "Same," and Jonah adds, "Maybe a week, or a little less."

Joey, the newbie in the ward, seems to drift in, and more often out of the conversation. It is obvious they're giving him massive amounts of meds; they must think he's at high risk of self-injury. I just hope ECT isn't in his future. Dinner is over. I take Kerin aside and tell her that I need a favor from her, a big favor. She shouldn't feel obligated, but I would appreciate her at least entertaining the idea.

She knows that I'm planning an epic show, and that I had hired an up-and-coming opera singer.

I propose, "I thought it might make it twice as good to have a duet. Would you consider being the second singer, with equal billing, of course?"

She is stunned, opens her eyes wide, and says, "Hell, yes, but my moms have to come."

"Deal," I add gleefully.

Back to my room, where there's just enough time to prepare two mochas before tonight's box of chocolates.

WASPy Ernie is the first up. He's been busy and updates me on how things are going with *Newton's Balls.* The balls are still in transit. I joke, "On the slow boat from China?"

No, he tells me they are being held up in customs at the Port of Los Angeles, which is the largest port of entry into the US from China.

They've never seen anything like eight-inch nickel-coated chrome steel ball bearings before and don't know what the hell they would be used for.

Ernie's tried to get in touch with the gas guy in South Boston, with no luck.

He shrugs. "He'll only speak to you."

I figure that the *Rising Snowflakes* and *Silver Pillows* will have to wait until my release.

Ernie takes his leave just as Lovely Wife arrives. A significant milestone has been reached: the *Fan Blowing Up Marilyn's Dress* project is done—put a fork in it. Our friend Keith has everything figured out: The grate is mounted in a box and a fan in the box blows the air up, and even better, Lovely Wife has been busy ordering a dozen white Marilyn gowns in various sizes and a bunch of blond wigs. She dropped off a couple of gowns and wigs with Keith, who reported that the test run went well: "All systems are go; we are ready for launch."

I am a bit obsessed with my release, but Lovely Wife has not heard anything specific about my expected release date. If things work out, it should be at the end of my second week, August 15. However, they won't give her a definite answer, just an "It depends." I plan to use my remaining time here to take notes for my book. It will both fulfill my promise to the Good One to do something of great importance and be my revenge.

It may take a while. However, as Eugène Sue so deliciously wrote in the text *Memoirs of Matilda* in the mid-1800s, "Revenge is a dish best served cold." Yet, I want my cold dish to be reheated by the sunlight—both the sunlight I hope to shine on mental health treatment and the sunlight I was denied here for too long. I'm done for the day and head straight to bed. Before dozing off, I think that maybe I can make a difference. No, scratch that. I will make a difference.

CHAPTER 13

"IT WAS A BRILLIANT CURE, BUT THE PATIENT DIED"

DAY 11: FRIDAY AUGUST 10

I'm up at 6:30 a.m., follow my usual routine, and then head to breakfast with Jonah. Kerin and Chief are there. Chief is looking sullen; he's scheduled for his third ECT treatment and typically sticks to juice. I grab my scrambled eggs, barista up my mocha, and join Kerin and Chief, with Jonah trailing close behind.

Kerin starts off excitedly, "I've picked the movie."

She grins at me, and I take the bait. "Okay, what is it?"

"*Pitch Perfect*."

I should have known. My head feels clearer now, possibly because the medical team is scaling back on my meds. More likely, it's due to my focusing on a purpose larger than myself: improving the mental health experience for the patients. It's time to put pedal to the metal.

I realize that since gaining phone privileges, I haven't reached out to anyone—no calls, texts, or emails. I've only used it for looking stuff up on the Internet. However, time is short, and I have to get directly involved with the people who are going to bring my show to life. No more middle-persons. I have to start connecting directly with the gang.

On the way back to my room after the movie, I stop to take my meds and head to the cafeteria for my real cure: the magic mocha. I notice a couple of the other patients doing the same. Word has spread, and knowing I've nudged some of them in the direction of imbibing a nontrivial mood enhancer makes me feel good. I can skip having my vitals checked, as they discontinued that routine a few days ago. Half an hour before lunch, back in my room, and being curious, I Google "caffeine and depression."

The first result that pops up is a study by Liu et al. titled "Low Dose of Caffeine Enhances the Efficacy of Antidepressants in Major Depressive Disorder," published in *Molecular Nutrition and Food Research,* 2017. The title says it all, but the article goes on to state, "The addition of caffeine may, by itself, reverse the development of depression and improve cognitive function." The beautiful part is that whether the findings are real or just a statistical anomaly, it doesn't matter. If you believe it's true—as I do—the placebo effect kicks in and makes it true.

Just then, Jonah shouts, "Lunch!" and off we go.

We grab the usual turkey sandwiches and head for the table where Joey, the new kid, is sitting with Kerin.

He appears sullen and relays, "I enjoyed being with you guys yesterday, but I've been feeling down. My mother tried to cheer me up by saying I am getting a 'special' treatment later today that the doctors told her should help me quite a bit."

Later today? I thought the treatments were administered in the morning. Just then, Chief shows up, explaining the situation. The ECT treatment center had "technical" difficulties yesterday, resulting in a backlog. As a result, he and Joey's treatments have been pushed back. Since today is Friday, and doctors don't work weekends, they have to get everyone done today.

The phrase "special" treatment," as used by Joey's mom, gets me thinking about Dana Carvey. I have been a fan of *Saturday Night Live* from the beginning. One episode I'll never forget was Carvey playing the Church Lady, who used her moralistic demeanor to describe a guest's questionable behavior with a condescending "Well, isn't that special?" Then, she accused them of being under the influence of "SATAN."

As we leave lunch, Chief and Joey look justifiably forlorn. They face ECT this afternoon, third time for Chief and first for Joey. I know I have to reassure them, once again, so I tell them, "Stay positive—it'll be okay."

I don't really believe this, but it does remind me that Norman Vincent Peale may have had it right with his influential, five-million-copy, best-selling 1952 book, *The Power of Positive Thinking*.

However, it's worth noting that Pastor Peale had his own dark side. He led the clergy in opposing the election of John F. Kennedy, not for his violation of the Seventh Commandment, "Thou shall not commit adultery," but rather because Kennedy was a Catholic.

Here we go again. Joey will have a much better chance of a positive outcome if he believes the treatment will have a positive outcome. If I assure him it will help, then the actual result of the treatment becomes less relevant than the benefits of the placebo effect. Conversely, if I tell him it's all bullshit and the side effects are dreadful, guess what? The placebo's evil twin, the nocebo effect comes into play. The nocebo effect occurs when negative outcomes result from the belief that a treatment will cause harm.

As the others leave, I stay behind at the table, reflecting on my now frequent ethical conundrum. I genuinely believe that ECT is a barbaric, harmful treatment. Yet, paradoxically, by lying and saying it will help, it probably will. Abracadabra, like magic, a lie becomes the truth. Placebos, nocebos, and lies—oh, my! It's becoming overwhelming; my head is about to explode.

I grab a couple of coffees and several packs of Nestlé, then head back to the room with Jonah to get ready for the daily outing. I make a mental note to self: ensure Joey is on the list for tomorrow. Jonah mentions that his parents, twin sister, and ex-girlfriend are visiting tonight and would like to spend a few minutes with me. My first thought is that it might be some kind of intervention; perhaps I'm a bad influence on their son. Less likely, they would like to meet me since Jonah has described me as a charming, witty, kind, and most crucially, empathetic guy . . . ha. In any event, I'll comb my hair. I assure Jonah that "I'd love to meet the family."

We head off to the great beyond. No matter how many times I navigate the labyrinth to the outside world, I become totally disoriented. I also wonder why the hell it's here. Who designed this thing? Clearly an afterthought at best, or an intentional, cruel joke. Eventually, the door at the end opens, and we're back in the gym. Yesterday's game was disappointing.

Despite placing the two best players, Kerin and Chief, on opposing teams and splitting up Jonah and me, no one else managed to score. Passes to other teammates resulted in fumbles or kicking the ball out of bounds—some actually believed we were playing soccer. Being good sports, none of the four of us tried to score. Mercifully, the game ended zero–zero, when Jason blew his whistle.

Today, we are returning to fundamentals: dribbling and passing drills. We begin with passing, which, unsurprisingly, is a complete "debacle," the French term for "fiasco," which is the Italian term for "failure." No matter the language, it isn't pretty. No one can catch or throw the ball, not underhand, not overhand—it's almost as if they have no hands.

So, I change it up. We all stand in a circle and hand the ball to the person on our left.

This continues smoothly until the next-to-last person literally drops the ball. Not bad. Whistle blows, and it's time to go outside. We decide to be Zen again today, no talking, just living for the moment. It puts you in a happy place, at least for me. Separating our consciousness from the distractions, constraints, and occasional cruelty of the physical world.

It takes me back to my marathon-running days. Roughly ten miles into a race, I'd separate my mind from my body and go into autopilot. Just to clarify, NOT Elon Musk's autopilot, which can cause bodily harm, but an autopilot where you just glide along. My mind would hover over and move along with my body. Periodically, I'd touch base with my body to see how things were going.

Most of the time, issues are manageable. However, after hitting the twenty-mile mark, your systems start to break down. Pain is actually feedback; it's data. It's the body's way of telling your brain how the rest of your body is doing. At this point, you have to turn off the autopilot to avoid serious damage. You go through a mental checklist: How are the legs doing, especially the calves, hamstrings, and quads?

Regardless of the answers, you suck it up, tough it out, and hopefully reach the finish line—of course, with both hands raised and looking up into the camera with a smile. A photo to show your grandchildren that Pop was once a contender. Although if Lovely Wife is at the viewing, she would add Forrest Gump's wise words, "Stupid is as stupid does." We complete our loop, smell the flowers, and head back to the reality of the ward.

In my room, I pivot to planning a different show. Since the *Defying Gravity* show has been delayed, September 5 is now open. It is Lovely Wife's birthday, and I'm orchestrating a surprise extravaganza for the twenty-seventh celebration of her thirty-ninth. Since September 5 is only a few weeks away, it's crunch time. I call my daughter, who has a knack for these things, to book a restaurant from 6:00 to 8:00 p.m. on the special day.

Fortunately, she has two phones. While talking to me on one, she texts one of her favorite restaurants with the other. She receives an affirmative and instructs me to call the restaurant and give them a $1,500 deposit. She suggests we opt for hors d'œuvres, a seventeenth-century French term derived from the Middle Age French word *entremets*, which basically means not a real meal.

In addition, there'll be an open bar so guests can drink and talk with friends while someone in an ill-fitting uniform passes around an unrecognizable tiny bite on a round platter. Since Emmett believes he's performing on September 5, it shouldn't be a problem for him. However, I realize that I haven't notified him that the *Defying Gravity* show has been rescheduled to October 30, the day before Halloween. I hope he can make it; I'll find out soon.

I text Emmett and ask when he can talk. Right away, I see the three dancing dots followed by "Now is good for me." I ask him how things are going, and he tells me that offers are pouring in. He's got a couple of upcoming opera roles in Germany, along with the Austin Opera Company.

Thinking to myself, I'm screwed, I stammer, "Umm, Emmett, there's been a change in plans. I have a medical issue and have to move the show back to October 30th. The venue is lined up, and I understand if you are booked."

He says, "One minute. Let me check my calendar."

A brief pause, then he responds, "No way I'm missing this. My mom's birthday is the next day, and she can't wait to see the show. I'm performing in San Francisco, but I'll catch the red-eye flight on the day of the show then fly out the next day."

Relieved, I say, "Thanks."

He quickly adds, "No problem. You paid me more than I asked for and paid in advance. Nobody has ever done that before. Thank you."

I decide to drop the other shoe. "About September 5th?"

"Of course," he responds. "I still have that circled on my calendar."

After a brief pause, I continue, "That's Lovely Wife's thirty-ninth birthday, and I'm throwing a surprise party. You'd just need to sing 'Happy Birthday' and do your Figaro number. I'll pay well."

Emmett replies, "Just cover my pianist. As for my payment, a kiss from the birthday girl will suffice."

"Deal. One last thing: I've come across an incredibly talented young soprano, Kerin, who trained at the Boston Conservatory at Berklee. I think she would be a great addition to the show."

Emmett interrupts me, "I love performing with sopranos. We can each do a solo, and then perform a couple of duets."

Wondering about the logistics, I ask, "Given the tight schedule, how will you two practice together?"

Emmett reassures me, "I'm good on the fly, and professionals are professional. I'll handle the pianist and getting a piano."

Good thing—I had completely forgotten about that part.

I walk past Kerin's room, and she's there. Having learned my lesson about NEVER entering someone else's room, I wave her into the hall.

"I have a proposal for you. Let's discuss it in the activity room," I offer.

She looks perplexed but curious. We walk to the empty activity room and sit at a small table in the corner.

I begin, "How would you like to perform at my show in New York City at the end of October?"

She lets out an excited shriek, then asks, "Will you cover the airfare for my moms and me?"

I nod. "Not only that, but I'll also reserve two hotel rooms and a stipend for you."

I go on to explain that she will be singing alongside a baritone.

"Does he have a name?" she inquires with a playful grin.

"Emmett O'Hanlon," I reply.

Kerin exclaims, "Holy shit! He's, like, famous. He almost won the Plácido Domingo's Operalia Competition last year." She continues, "I can't wait. In fact, give me his number, and we can figure out what we're going to sing."

Kerin explains that performing at a concert requires lead time. Unlike singing in the ward, tuning her "instrument" for a major event is a lengthy process.

"I have a big voice," she declares.

I smile. She comes across every inch the diva.

I'm feeling pretty good about what I've accomplished so far today. Not only finalizing the details for Lovely Wife's birthday party on September 5, but I also nailed down the singing portion of *Defying Gravity.* Pun alert: It feels like the weight of the world has been lifted off my shoulders.

I see Chief in the hall, and he waves me over and relays, "My treatment is at three o'clock, and Joey's at four. He's really scared. I don't think I can say much to comfort him. Maybe you can give him one of your pep talks."

He points to where Joey is sitting, engrossed with a Rubik's Cube.

Approaching Joey, I query, "How long does it take you to solve it?"

Joey laughs. "At the world championships in China earlier this year, I did it in eleven seconds."

I'm stunned. "Holy shit, that must be a world record."

Joey shakes his head. "No, just top twenty-five. Nobody can beat Yusheng Du; he did it in 3.47 seconds."

I follow up with, "How is that even possible?"

He explains, "You get really focused and drift into this other place where time slows down. It's hard to explain, but all the top players experience it. I play with the Cube to calm myself. My thoughts sometimes jump around. My happy place is spinning the cube."

I reassure him that everything is going to be okay, silently wondering if he'll even be able to solve the Cube after his "treatment."

Jonah and I head to dinner and find Kerin already there, seated at our table with a big smile. Chief and Joey are absent, recovering from their treatments. We grab our plates and join her. Uncharacteristically, I stay quiet, preoccupied with my to-do list. Why do I say "uncharacteristically"? I recall an interview I gave to a local newspaper about fifteen years ago.

A Boston newspaper was covering the story of my son's and my upcoming climb of Mount Kilimanjaro to raise money for cancer research. My brother had recently lost a battle to an unusually lethal cancer of unknown origin. It was likely the result of significant Agent Orange exposure in the Vietnam War. Despite the bleak prognosis, a research scientist at Beth Israel Hospital provided my brother with hope. This scientist, renowned for his pioneering work using zebrafish—their transparency makes them ideal for observing cancer growth—would be the beneficiary of the funds raised.

We set a goal of one dollar for each foot of elevation: 19,430. The article was quite positive, but there was one adjective the journalist used to describe me with which I was unfamiliar—loquacious. I looked it up and found it is derived from the Latin word *loquax*, which means "talkative." Of course, I was, and am, just not right now at the table.

Jonah is also quiescent, no doubt thinking about his family's imminent visit. On the flip side, Kerin is stoked. She's reached out to the Boston Conservatory for assistance with her arrangement, shared her plans with her moms (who are not totally on board yet), and begun voice and breathing exercises. She's busy curating her look: the gown, shoes, makeup, lipstick, earrings, and necklace. She is starting to sound like my daughter getting ready for prom; yes, she did attend prom, several of them. But then again, she didn't score 800 on her math SAT—just 740.

Jonah gets word of his family's arrival and turns to me, saying, "Let's go. It's showtime."

In the hallway, I spot four people, his parents (presumably) and two young women. It's hard for me to tell which one is his twin sister, and which is his ex-girlfriend. We exchange introductions and settle into the activity room, which is, fortunately, empty.

We gather at a table, and Jonah's mother begins, "We all want to express our profound gratitude. Jonah has told us how wonderful it is to be with you and the sense of hope and purpose you've instilled in him; we all can feel it. Over the past year or so, he has felt that he has let everyone down, especially himself. We've assured him this isn't true. However, sometimes the action of an outsider can speak louder than our words."

She continues, "He hasn't stopped talking about the event, how you trusted him to organize things and order all the food. He couldn't resist smiling when he told us how you'd rather give everyone a positive experience even at the risk of facing the consequences. You just wanted people to have some fun. He views you as a role model, and for that, we are grateful. Finally, you have given us hope for his future. Thank you."

She ends it there, and I'm left thinking what she really means is, "Since you've reached the ripe old age of sixty-five, maybe there's hope for Jonah." I wonder what's so extraordinary about reaching my age. However, it's understandable that parents of younger adults with bipolar disorder have genuine concerns. I Googled it, and unfortunately, it's hard to unsee the first hit: "Patients with bipolar disorder live thirteen years less than their healthy peers."

I stand up and thank them for their kind words. I convey that I've greatly benefited from my time with Jonah and the rest of the ward, adding, "Jonah is a very talented young man with a good heart; he's going to do well. Above all, Jonah and the other patients have given me a purpose that I've been seeking for a while."

They are all smiles as I bid them . . . adieu.

Exiting the room, I spot Lovely Wife waiting. We head off to our usual rendezvous spot in the hallway. For some reason, we always meet there, probably a vestige of when I was committed to the high-security section of the ward and could only converse across the DMZ. For those unfamiliar, DMZ stands for demilitarized zone, a reference to the barrier separating North and South Korea after the Korean War, which could not be crossed.

Excited, Lovely Wife recounts her encounter with Jeremy's parents and twin sister in the parking lot.

Befuddled, I ask, "You mean Jonah? I've heard about a third twin, but I've never spoken to a Jeremy."

She clarifies, "He's the tall, skinny boy with a twin sister—Jeremy."

And in a hushed voice, Lovely Wife adds, "His twin sister was speaking rapidly and seemed jittery. I suspect she has the 'gift' along with Jeremy."

Lovely Wife proceeds to describe the conversation she had with Jeremy's mother.

"She expressed how grateful she was for your efforts to improve life on the ward."

Referring to the party, Jeremy's mom asked, "How did he manage that? It's the only positive thing Jeremy has mentioned about his stay at MrClean."

Lovely Wife replied, "He hates rules and always finds a way around them. He's still a child."

"Actually, we found it reassuring to see a 'mature' patient here."

So, once again, I'm an inspiration for having survived being crazy for all this time. I guess Paul Simon and I have that in common.

Shifting gears, she briefs me on *Newton's Balls*.

"Zach has some information and wants you to call tomorrow morning before nine."

"Good news or bad news?"

"Well, he seemed pretty excited, so I'm betting on good news."

Perplexed, I ask her why everyone treats her as the gatekeeper for my contact with the outside world.

She explains, "At first, you didn't have a phone, so I was the only way to reach you. Later, they just preferred interacting with me."

My riposte: "Touché," a French term used in fencing to acknowledge a hit by one's opponent, and commonly used as a nod to another person's clever point in a verbal exchange.

She has grandson duties awaiting her, so she bids me a preemptive . . . adieu, and I parry with another "Touché."

I head back to my room to read the book I had asked Lovely Wife to bring: Hemingway's *The Old Man and the Sea*. The narrative resonates with my newfound identity: "the Old Man." Released at the same time in *Life* magazine and as a Charles Scribner's Sons book on September 1, 1951, the novella is a succinct 140 pages and 28,704 words. Averaging 500 words a day, Hemingway completed it in about eight weeks. He had a huge return on the time invested: The magazine issue sold out five million copies in two days, with fifty thousand copies of the first edition of the book snapped up soon thereafter.

My connection to Hemingway's Old Man goes back many years. A decade ago, I attempted to purchase a first edition at the Shakespeare and Company in Paris's fifth arrondissement. Suspecting my tendency toward hypomania's excessive spending even then, Lovely Wife gave me a hard NO. She argued that fifteen hundred dollars for a used book was absurd, and suggested I buy the paperback for $10.99 on Amazon instead. She finished her tirade with, "It's the same story." So, I complied. That very copy I am now holding. However, without undermining her victory, that same first edition is now selling for four thousand dollars on AbeBooks.

Hemingway won the Nobel Prize in literature in 1954 primarily for *The Old Man and the Sea*, and was recognized for "his mastery of the art of narrative." This was the last major work he published during his lifetime. After that, Hemingway appeared adrift. He began multiple new projects but failed to complete them. He even felt he was being followed, which his friends brushed off as paranoia. However, years later, it was revealed that J. Edgar Hoover did indeed have him under surveillance in Havana for many years. His mental health spiraled downward, and he was checked into the Mayo Clinic for "hypertension." That was a guise; he was actually being treated for severe depression. The treatment involved—wait for it—a shocking FIFTEEN rounds of electroconvulsive shock treatment.

Afterward, he asked his friend A. E. Hotchner, "What is the sense of ruining my head and erasing my memory, which is my capital, and putting me out of business? It was a brilliant cure, but we lost the patient."

I'll let that sink in . . . his body remained alive, but his soul was dead. Shortly thereafter, he received three additional rounds of ECT at the Mayo Clinic. Three months later, on July 2, 1961, at the age of sixty-one, he returned to his family home in Ketchum, Idaho. He took his beloved Abercrombie & Fitch shotgun, placed it in his mouth, and pulled the trigger.

Hemingway was gone by sixty-one. Now I understand why everyone here is inspired by my longevity. Ernest and I likely share the same disease; we're bipolar twins, except I've outlived him by four years. Am I living on borrowed time? I haven't given much thought to my age before. The first milestone I recall was turning sixteen and being able to drive. At eighteen, I could both drink legally and be drafted. By nineteen, Congress had ratified the Twenty-Sixth Amendment, and I could vote. At twenty-five, I could rent a car. Thirty was a notable threshold, after which, according to Jack Weinberg's 1964 maxim, I could no longer be trusted. He wasn't just a clever linguist but the catalyst for a student activation movement resulting from his arrest for setting up a table at Cal Berkeley to support free speech. Now fast-forward, and forty, fifty, or even sixty didn't faze me. But turning sixty-four was the first time I admitted that I might be old. Thanks to the Beatles.

Now I'm sixty-five, and now I'm asleep.

CHAPTER 14

"I HAVE TO LIE TO TELL THE TRUTH"

DAY 12: SATURDAY, AUGUST 11

I'm up at 6:00 a.m., and as I step into the hall, Jason is waiting with a towel. We head to the bathroom for my daily ritual. I then head back to the room, and, like a tag team, Jonah leaves for his daily morning ritual. At seven, we head to breakfast. Kerin is already seated at our usual table, but Chief and Joey are missing. They had their treatments late yesterday, so they're most likely sleeping in. We probably won't see them until lunch.

Out of the blue, Jonah remarks, "It's weird. Much of the group is getting ECT, and we somehow escaped it. It kind of makes sense for Kerin and me, since we're not in such bad shape, but you seem like the ideal target. Plus, management doesn't like you very much."

I smile. "Yeah, they kind of alluded to it. I think they realized that things could go really off the rails. ECT is supposed to turn you into a complacent automaton, but in my case, they were probably worried that it might have the opposite effect, and all hell would break loose. Less likely, they thought I was progressing nicely. Or maybe they believe I'm just a crazy know-it-all who hates authority, and instead of being treatment-resistant mentally ill, I'm just plain resistant."

We all laugh, and Kerin quickly adds, "You're not wrong about that. We all think you are crazy, but in a good way."

I forgot to pick up my phone from the "safe" central charging station, so I ask Jonah the time.

"Eight o'clock," he replies.

I'm wondering if it's too early to call Zach about the balls. Lovely Wife mentioned that he was "excited." If it were me, I'd be up. I take my leave. In the hallway, I grab my cellphone and realize that I don't have Zach's number, so I text Lovely Wife. After fifteen agonizing minutes, she texts me his number. She's not thrilled that I pinged her a dozen times and used "Find her iPhone" twice, with that irritating repeating ding. As I may have mentioned, Lovely Wife is not a morning person and dislikes being disturbed, to put it mildly.

At this point, the meds have turned my short-term memory to mush, and I can't remember the number long enough to dial it. I've got nothing to write with, and the crayons are locked in the activity room until 10:00. I'm flummoxed. Then I notice the phone number in the text is underlined, reminding me that I can dial by tapping it.

One of the wonders of the modern world, right up with remote controls, automatic garage door openers, and Japanese toilets: I tap the number, and the call connects. After three rings, I usually hang up, assuming the other person has better things to do than talk to me. But this time, I wait. Zach picks up.

Out of breath, he exclaims, "They're on their way! The fucking balls are on their way. The customs guy loved the Newton's cradle I sent. It was one of his favorite toys as a kid, and he keeps one on his desk. He expedited things, and not only are the balls on the way, but he also arranged for quick shipment. Each of the fifteen balls weighs eighty pounds, and with the crate, the whole thing comes to fifteen hundred pounds. It's pricy to expedite the shipment, but regular freight takes a month."

"How much?" I inquire.

Zach replies, "Eleven thousand five hundred bucks, but they'll air ship and deliver right to my workshop in two days."

I respond, "No choice. Let's do it." Then as an afterthought, "Don't tell Lovely Wife."

I then get ahold of Paul, the steel fabricator, to finalize the design of the cradle part of *Newton's Balls*.

I summarize my concept, and Paul offers, "Sounds good. I'd say twenty-five thousand dollars for the parts. Labor's on me."

I respond, "Thanks. Go for it."

All in, *Newton's Balls* will cost just over $100,000—a bargain for the world's largest well-hung balls. Lovely Wife won't be the wiser—unless she reads this.

After my skipped lunch, I meet up with Kerin and Jonah. The three of us have successfully booked our "death row" hour of outdoor time. Even though it is a Saturday, we have an outing. Fortunately, outings don't take the weekends off. The nurses oversee this activity and operate on a rotating schedule, ensuring they are fully staffed 24/7. Doctors have little to do with these excursions. For some reason, they overlook the healing power of nature.

Jonah and I head for the rendezvous point, and Kerin is there waiting at the door. Chief and Joey are passing. Chief is really feeling the effects of three treatments in five days. Joey is reeling from his first. I'm feeling a mix of sympathy and anger. Actually, I'm beyond angry—I'm pissed off, really pissed off. I'll also throw in helpless. There's nothing I can do now except go along with the story line here that shock treatment is their best option. However, I will use my anger later when I am not helpless to tell the story.

As usual, a capacity crowd. We navigate through the various doors, down the stairs, and then enter the labyrinth that will lead us to the gym.

Before we get there, Debbie, a Minnesotan with an accompanying Midwest accent, sticks her head out from one of the offices in the labyrinth.

"Let's meet up later," she suggests.

I reply, "Sure," which is my shorthand for "I hope I never see you again."

Apparently, Debbie is my social worker, and I know she's planning to give me all those neuropsych tests that I find tedious and annoying, flea-bite annoying. I'll try to hold her off—hopefully forever—although she looks persistent.

Back to the labyrinth beneath MrClean Hospital's campus. We reach the door at the end of the hallway and enter the gym. Anticipating a repeat of yesterday's disaster, and given that Chief can't make it, I decide to start easy with the circle pass. I explain, once again, the game to the group. We form a circle and pass the basketball to the person on the left. I position Jonah to my left to ensure the first handoff is successful, and Kerin to my right so we don't fumble the last one if it makes it that far. This setup also has the benefit of having my two friends on either side of me. I pass the ball to Jonah, he hands it to the next person, and then, very slowly, we get the ball to the penultimate camper.

Shit, it's the girl who dropped the ball yesterday, who we've nicknamed Klutz, an Americanized version of the Yiddish word *klots*, meaning a clumsy person or blockhead. She grabs the ball, but then, instead of giving it to Kerin, hands it back to the person who gave it to her.

Kerin yells, "NO, pass me the ball!"

Klutz tries to retrieve the ball but fumbles it. We're all on edge at this point, but fortunately Kerin snatches it in midair and gives it to me. Victory! Some of us raise our "number one" index finger, some give a fist pump, others just smile, and a few just stare into the ether.

This is good therapy; a sense of accomplishment is infinitely better than the "treatments" they are administering here. After all, it's those treatments that are depriving Chief and Joey of this euphoric moment. The crucial question the mental health testing group should be asking is "Have you experienced happiness in the last two weeks?" For us, the answer is a resounding "Hell, yes. Both at the gym and at the PARTY." I sense another song coming on, one of the all-time bests. It's played at the end of every sport's championship game. We've earned it. To paraphrase Queen, "We are the champions—of the ward."

Energized, we venture out to the great beyond—where today, the "loons" are free to roam. Well, at least a little free. As has been our habit, Kerin, Jonah, and I form the nucleus of the fast group. In fact, today we ARE the fast group. Off we go.

During the walk, Kerin shares that she will be released in about a week. However, she won't be able to go home right away. She needs to spend time in a residential treatment facility in Tennessee.

"What's that?" I ask.

"It's like a halfway house, a transition for people they believe aren't ready to go home yet," she explains.

I ask her, "How does that make you feel?" (Note the empathy.)

"It sucks. What's worse, my moms say that I won't be able to return to Berklee to continue with my classical training. They think that the stress of singing, along with the competitions, was worsening my condition."

I quickly interrupt, "It's not an illness, Kerin. You are different. For you, it's a gift."

She smiles. "My moms also want me to spend some time at home, so that's where I'm headed after the residential program. Hey, I just got a thought: Maybe you can convince them that I should continue with my music. There's a joint program with MorAss General Hospital called the Berklee Music Therapy Program. They are doing innovative research and have early results that music can have amazing positive effects on the 'gift,' as you call it. I'd be the perfect choice; I've experienced both sides."

I respond, "I'll give it a shot," and notice I'm humming Joni Mitchell's "Both Sides Now."

Jonah interjects, with a broad smile, "Thanks again for seeing my family. They were on the fence about whether I should return to Brandeis at all. However, they've noticed good progress since I've been here and offered a compromise. If I take the fall semester off and get a job at the music store where I've worked before, they'll let me attend the spring semester. I'm stoked."

Perplexed, I query, "You worked in a music store?"

Jonah replies, "Yeah, I was in an electrotech band, a fusion of electronic and techno music styles. It suits me because I'm really good at playing electronic musical instruments but suck at singing. Fortunately, there are no vocals with the electrotech genre. I was really good at sales; I'd draw people into the store with my playing. Sometimes I'd gather a crowd, and they'd start jumping to the electrotech beat."

Kerin butts in, "Where was the store?"

Jonah answers, "The Guitar Center."

Kerin says, "Across from Berklee?"

"Yup."

Kerin continues, "I'd sometimes walk by there and would have to cross the street because, no offense, I hate that sound."

Jonah adds, "None taken."

We all laugh.

Now that we've discovered there are two bona fide musicians in our group, I unveil that I am a pioneer of a new genre of music. During one of my previous, undiagnosed manic episodes, my anger for our current president—who likely played a significant role in triggering said episode—unleashed a latent musical talent lurking deep within the neural clusters of my brain.

Just as the long-dormant prehistoric sea monster, Godzilla, was awakened in Japan by nuclear fallout, my inner Beethoven was awakened by rage-induced mania. In the span of fifteen minutes, I penned a song, downloaded GarageBand, figured out audio recording, sang my song, then uploaded it to Spotify. Since it contained both gospel and rap elements, I naturally named the genre gospel rap. When my smarty-pants Harvard Law School niece heard about it, she sniped, "Gospel rap? That's not a thing." Unbeknownst to her, her quip was pure genius. I now had the name for my album to follow: *Gospel Rap. It's Not a Thing*. I got nine downloads, three of them mine.

Mercifully, Kerin changes the subject. "By the way, are you still getting out on Wednesday?"

I answer, "I haven't heard anything to the contrary."

Both Kerin and Jonah chime in, "We'll miss you."

I say, "I'll definitely see Kerin when she sings at my New York City event, and Jonah, I'll be at Brandeis next spring. They're teaching my case, and you can be my guest."

We reach the end of our walk and stop to appreciate the flowers—maybe even taking a whiff or two—before heading back to the ward.

As unluck would have it, halfway back through the labyrinth, I encounter not the Minotaur, but even worse—social worker Debbie. She blocks my path and informs me that I will be taking my tests tomorrow at 1:00 p.m.

When I ask how long it will take, she responds, "About an hour."

I let her know, "I have my mandated one-hour outdoor time tomorrow starting at 1:30 p.m., so let's start at 12:20 p.m."

She begrudgingly agrees, a decision which, no doubt, will cut into her lunch "hour."

The group pauses for me since the guiding principle here is "Leave no crazy behind," and we make our way back to the ward. As I'm heading to my room, I learn that Chief and Joey are in the cafeteria waiting for me. It's 2:30 p.m., so I can "skin two cats with one knife": comfort Joey and Chief and prepare my magic mocha. I dislike the expression "Kill two birds with one stone," since I love birds with their grace and ability to fly and dislike cats, since they prey on birds.

I walk over to the table where Joey and Chief are sitting and tell them I will be right back. They nod, understanding my caffeine ritual. I've streamlined the process by skipping the step of heating the coffee to 145 degrees Fahrenheit after pouring it into the cup as the microwave sometimes has a queue. Instead, I pour in the Nestlé cocoa, add the hot coffee, stir, and drink. The coffee is usually hot enough, and if not, I wait for the microwave.

Sometimes when I do end up waiting in line, just for fun, I ask a fellow inmate standing in front of me if they think it's possible to leave a metal spoon in the microwave.

They inevitably respond, "No way. Everyone knows it'll catch fire or explode."

I challenge, "You wanna bet?"

The easy mark retorts, "Yeah, how much?"

I reply, "The loser has to cluck like a chicken for five seconds."

The unsuspecting patsy usually agrees, saying, "You're on."

So, I take my coffee, put a metal spoon in, and set the microwave for thirty seconds. A small crowd gathers around, standing at a safe distance. I put my face right up against the glass as the crowd murmurs, "He's fucking crazy." High praise considering the source. Am I left disfigured for life when it explodes in my face? No. Nothing happens except my coffee heats up.

Puzzled voices echo, "Huh."

Perhaps unsurprisingly, most of my victims actually do cluck like a chicken, some flapping their arms.

I return to the table and ask Joey and Chief how they're doing.

Joey begins, "I have a terrible headache, and I can't remember much. I'm having trouble holding on to a thought. It's scary."

Chief interjects, "The fatigue is the worst for me. I used to work out for three hours—no problem. Now I get tired just sitting up."

He continues, "Plus, I get really disoriented. I often don't know the time of day, who's scheduled to visit—whether it's my parents, brother, friends, or coach."

I remind him that his parents and brother are scheduled for tonight.

"Yeah, that's right, and they want to meet you."

I know the answer to my next question, "So, you guys skipped lunch?"

Joey says, "I felt really sick to my stomach," and Chief says, "I about just threw up thinking about it."

How did I know? I Googled it. Nausea is the number one side effect of ECT, according to the Mayo Clinic.

Joey asks, "Are you sure this is the best treatment?"

Chief chimes in, "Yeah, after each session I feel as bad or worse than the previous one. It feels like I'm heading in the wrong direction. So, what's the deal? Is this really helping? Will it make us better?"

I'm really starting to hate that question. Once again, I am caught between the proverbial rock and a hard place. I know what to say.

"Look, we're all here because we need help. Our loved ones really care and want the best for us. They've sent us to the top psychiatric hospital in the country. The doctors here are among the world's leading psychiatrists and neuroscientists. They think ECT is the gold standard treatment. So, if they believe it, then we should as well."

Do I actually say that? No fucking way. They would nod off at the "Our loved ones" part, maybe me too. So, what do I say? A one-word answer: "Yes." To which they both respond with nods. I cling to the hope this will maintain the placebo effect, which I still believe is their best shot. I have to continue down that path. After all, what choice do I have? I don't want to become "that" guy, Mr. Nocebo. So, once again, I have to lie to tell the truth.

We spend the rest of the afternoon sitting mostly in silence. I think Joey and Chief are happy to have the company of a father figure, almost a grandfather figure. After a while, they chase us out to get the cafeteria ready for another gourmet meal.

I skip arts and crafts today; hopefully I won't be dinged. I retreat to my room for a much-needed nap; the silent company of Joey and Chief was surprisingly exhausting.

Jonah eventually wakes me up, and we head to the cafeteria for dinner. I'm not overly concerned about getting there early since I have decided to have the fish tonight. Why the fish, you might ask? Simple—it's the law of diminishing marginal utility, a concept I frequently encountered when I was studying to be a quantitative economist. After ten scoops of your favorite ice cream, let's say chocolate, you'd prefer something different, like vanilla.

So much for theory. The fish sucked—absolutely inedible, and projectile-vomit bad. I've had turkey for eleven nights in a row, but the law of decreasing marginal utility doesn't seem to have kicked in yet. I should never have chosen the fish. I discovered it has negative marginal utility, which means I would pay money to not eat it.

Jonah and I head back to our room to do a little reading before visiting hour. Tonight, it's Jack Kerouac's *On the Road*, which I found in the activity room. It's considered the defining book of the pre-hippie movement, known as the Beat Generation. *The New York Times* labeled it a masterpiece. I was a bit surprised to see it here, given that it is the quintessential antiestablishment book. The innocuous, all-American title must have misled the hospital censors. I had read it many years ago, and its backstory is legendary. Kerouac wrote the book while living in Manhattan, on a single 120-foot scroll that he made by taping together sheets of tracing paper. He completed the ninety-thousand-word book in three weeks, hardly sleeping and fueled by pea soup and Benzedrine. The original scroll sold in 2001 for $2.43 million to Jim Irsay, a rich guy who also owned the Indianapolis Colts.

Now for the bad news. After skimming the book for about half an hour, I realize that the backstory is far more interesting than the book itself. Even though I can identify with the sidekick, Neal Cassady, who is clearly manic and Bipolar I, I wish they'd cut the road trip short. Cassady is a world-class prankster, but I'd rather pull off a prank than read about someone else's.

I hear Kerin in the hallway. "Chief's parents and brother are here."

I respond, "On it."

I wander out into the hallway, and at the end by the nurse's station stands a group of large people. One looks just like Chief, so that's obviously his twin brother. Wait a minute, which one is Chief? Oh yeah, the one in pajamas. Interestingly, Chief's brother is smiling and appears to not share Chief's condition. His father, equally large and equally fit, is wearing a tight-fitting T-shirt, his biceps about the size of my calf muscles—and I have big calves.

Chief's mom looks pretty buff as well, sporting her Lululemon yoga pants. We shake hands, and I do my best not to cringe in pain as they apply a viselike grip, Chief's mother included.

At this point, Kerin appears, grabs Chief, and says, "I'll take Ben to get a snack in the cafeteria and give you guys a chance to talk."

I suggest we move to the activity room for our conversation.

Ben's mom begins by explaining the family's concerns about Ben over the last six months.

"Ever since his injury stopped his training, he has gone into a funk—no, worse than that, a depression. It began after his wrestling season ended and got progressively worse. We took him to a doctor, who prescribed several different medications, but Ben's condition continued to deteriorate. That doctor referred us to another, who then recommended a third, each one prescribing different medications. The last doctor advised, 'Due to the trajectory of his depression, we think he should be admitted to a hospital.' That's how he ended up here."

She adds, "When they proposed electroconvulsive shock treatment, we were terrified. We thought they didn't do that anymore, but the hospital assured us it was his best option, referring to it as the 'gold standard.'"

"Ah, yes," I say to myself. "The good old 'gold standard.'"

"Anyway, we want to thank you for looking after him. Ben mentioned that you've been instrumental in making his stay here tolerable, especially with his adverse reaction to the treatment. He also mentioned you believed it will help him. Is that true?"

Uh-oh, I'm cornered. At this point, I'm sure my Pinocchio nose has grown six inches. Do I tell them what I really think, that ECT might work for its placebo effect but seems more like a form of nineteenth-century torture? No, expressing my real feelings wouldn't help Ben. By revealing skepticism, it would undermine their confidence in the procedure. Instilling doubt in their minds could inadvertently put doubt in Ben's mind, thus undermining the proven power of positive thinking. Following my script, I assure them that doctors consider ECT "the gold standard" and believe in its efficacy. Once again, I resort to a lie to allow the magic of the placebo effect to turn into actual healing.

Giving me a taboo hug, I bid them all . . . adieu.

I head back to my room, grab a coffee and a Nestlé packet, head to the cafeteria, and do my mocha thing. As I exit, Lovely Wife excitedly heads over.

"Zach got a call: The balls have arrived at Logan Airport and will be delivered to Paul's shop by noon tomorrow," she announces.

I respond, "That's great, but why didn't he call me directly?"

Lovely Wife replies, "He doesn't feel comfortable calling you since he's afraid he might be interrupting something important."

I retort, "What can be more important than the balls?"

She laughs and adds, "Maybe he just likes me better." Amen to that.

She continues, "The Tesla has been delivered, and they're anxious for you pick it up. I've told them you're tied up (as in a straitjacket, ha ha) but assured them you'll be there on Wednesday before four o'clock. You'll need proof of insurance and a certified check before they hand over the car. I'll get those tomorrow and bring them to you, but please don't lose them. If you don't pick the car up on Wednesday, it goes to the next person on the list, and you'll go to the back of what is now a three-month wait."

I reply, "Okay, no problem."

I'm thinking that Elon Musk is the "Car Nazi." Take too much time, and it's "No car for you." He also appears as bipolar as they come, minimal sleep, grandiosity, hypersexual, and on and on. He may not even know that he and Kanye West have become the poster children for the disorder, showcasing both the genius and destructive tendencies that come with being bipolar.

She glances at her watch and announces she has to go. As she turns to leave, she adds, "Oh, by the way, I brought something for you," and hands me a stack of unlined paper and a small contraband pen. "I want you to write another chapter for your book. I know you need deadlines, so if it's not done by tomorrow, no Tesla for you."

I'm pretty sure she's joking, but she is right. I'd forgotten about my book project, soon to be a Netflix series, at least that's what manic me believes. It was to be my first book, but now it will be a number two. I'll work on it tomorrow.

I head back to my room, smiling to myself. I can't believe she is going to let me pick up the Tesla and drive it twenty miles home. I have no clue how to operate it, but I know it can go zero to sixty in three seconds—just as quick as the Rock 'n' Roller Coaster at Disney World. I'm sure the bipolar Elon did that on purpose. There's no way I'm not testing that out.

Just as I step into my room, I hear Kerin tuning up her voice with Schubert's 1825 masterpiece, "Ave Maria." Its transcendent beauty resonates through the halls.

I glance over and see Jonah is engrossed in his book *Advanced Python*. You might ask, "Is that a book about an exceptionally smart snake?" Well, it's not. Actually, Python is currently the leading computer programming language. Kids like Jonah consider Fortran and Cobol, which I used in the 1970s, to be ancient languages. I bet they're unaware of the stack of punch cards you needed to feed through the computer to run the programs.

But where did Guido van Rossum, the creator of the Python programming language, come up with the name? Guido recalls that during the 1989 Christmas holidays, he was engrossed in the published scripts of the BBC comedy series *Monty Python's Flying Circus*, which featured six young British comedians. At the same time, he was also writing a new programming language that needed a name. Suddenly he had an epiphany: He liked the show's name and truncated it to "Python," deeming it "slick," like a snake.

However, this begs the question: How did *Monty Python's Flying Circus* get its name in the first place? Legend has it that the "Monty" part was a mocking tribute to Field Marshal Lord Montgomery, a renowned British

World War II general. "Python" was added to imply Monty was also a snake. So, indeed, the name Advanced Python does have its roots in a snake.

I still have an hour before I need to return my phone to the charging station. They've devised a simple yet effective strategy to ensure we return our phones on time. On a table near the central command—where the nurses and attendants are stationed—there's a large docking station with twenty-two charging ports, each labeled with a room number.

Phones plug directly into these ports without any cords required, eliminating another choking hazard. For those without phones, their port is marked with an unremovable "no phone" sticker. If your phone isn't docked by 9:00 p.m., the staff will track you down and confiscate your phone until your discharge day. It's very effective and makes me wonder why they don't use that clever thinking to develop more humane ways to treat the patients.

Before my time expires (bad choice of words), I have a couple of questions to ask my friend Google. I've noticed that our ward has three sets of twins, which seems suspiciously high. Is there a correlation between being a twin and being bipolar? More generally, how significant are genetics in determining mental differences—specifically bipolar disorder, my specialty? According to Google, research shows that 3.3 percent (or one in thirty) of the general population is bipolar. However, if one parent has the condition, the chances rise to 20 percent (one in five) that a given child of theirs will also have it. If both parents are bipolar, the odds double to 40 percent (two in five). The rates are the same for females and males.

Now, on to twins. In the case of fraternal twins, where two eggs are fertilized—pretentious scientists refer to this as dizygotic—the likelihood of either twin being bipolar is independent of the other, the same as if they were ordinary siblings. In other words, if neither parent is bipolar, there's a 3.3 percent chance that the first fraternal twin will be bipolar. Furthermore, if the first fraternal twin is bipolar, the odds of the second fraternal twin being bipolar are the same 3.3 percent. The likelihood of both being bipolar is 0.1 percent (one in nine hundred).

For identical or monozygotic twins, the story is very different. If one identical twin is bipolar, the other has at least an 80 percent chance of being bipolar. Identical twins are inherently linked; what happens to one will most likely happen to the other, as if they were . . . identical. That is not surprising, since they share the exact same DNA.

This brings me to the much-debated question in medicine: "Is being bipolar mostly a product of the environment or genes?" Those who support the environmental hypothesis argue that a parent or parents who are bipolar might create a family environment where the actions and behaviors of the parent(s) imprints on the child(ren), which triggers them to mirror the bipolarity of the parent(s). On the flip side, geneticists argue that a person becomes bipolar exclusively due to their genes; in other words, the environment plays no role.

This question has been examined exhaustively, and the answer is, 80 percent genes and 20 percent environment. And the 20 percent might just represent something in the environment triggering a latent genetic trait. So, maybe it is 100 percent genetic. With a father and grandfather who were both bipolar, the odds were about one out of four that I would be bipolar. Yet, as it turned out, I beat the odds and won the bipolar lottery.

My phone indicates it's 8:58 p.m. I have two minutes to run to the charging station. I just make it. And yes, someone was there checking.

CHAPTER 15

"AREA 51"

DAY 13: SUNDAY, AUGUST 12

I bolt upright, wide awake. I look at the clock in the room, and it's 4:00 a.m. I remember Lovely Wife mentioning that I had to get going on the next chapter in my book. I hate procrastinating, and hate it even more when she reminds me I'm procrastinating. The drugs at MrClean have sapped me of my desire to write so far. But today is the day to fight back. I've been writing a series of short stories, all based on true events, which I plan to publish as a collection. The joke is that most readers will think they're fiction because you'd have to be crazy to actually do the things I describe. I've titled it *More Cowbell.* It's based on the *SNL* skit featuring Will Ferrell on cowbell and Christopher Walken as the band's producer. The song they are working on isn't working. Walken realizes it needs "more cowbell." The phrase is a metaphor for seeking more life in life. That is my mantra and my title.

I was inspired by six-foot, nine-inch, likely bipolar Michael Crichton's book *Travels* (1988). It consists of twenty-nine chapters with catchy titles such as "A Human Light Show," "Spoon Bending," "Seeing Headhunters," and "Climbing Kilimanjaro." Lovely Wife gave it to me about ten years ago and nonchalantly opined, "You will relate to this book; you could have written it." I took it as a compliment—after all, Crichton has written some of the greatest books of all time, with *Jurassic Park* being both epoch and epic.

However, what Lovely Wife really meant was that, like Crichton, I took excessive risks and pursued difficult challenges just for the hell of it. Crichton often got less than four hours of sleep when up against a self-imposed deadline. He was, in many ways, another poster child for Bipolar disorder, and Lovely Wife was hinting—not so subtly—that I belonged on that poster as well.

I should also credit Ernest Hemingway as a motivator for me to write that book.

Hemingway has always had a big impact on me. He inspired me to break out of the "status quo bias," the tendency for people to remain within their comfort zone. I joined his club, where members grab life by the throat and choke it until it reveals its innermost secrets.

Among his outlandish exploits was during World War II, when he led French Resistance fighters into liberated Paris after the Nazis were routed by the Allied forces in August 1944. While the Allied forces awaited an official "all clear" outside Paris, Hemingway grabbed a rifle, hopped in a tank, and led the somewhat sober Resistance fighters into the city. He marched straight to the Ritz Hotel and didn't leave until the alcohol ran out at the open bar. The most bizarre part? He wasn't even in the military—he was a war correspondent for *Collier's magazine*, yet no one seemed to notice.

He also penned *The Snows of Kilimanjaro* (1952), which not only compelled me to climb it but also to ascend via the most dangerous route, the dreaded Western Breach. Fewer than one in a hundred climbers attempt that route, yet over half the fatalities occur there. Upon a second reading, after my climb, I discovered, with a grin, that Hemingway never actually climbed it—he merely shot a Cape buffalo in its shadow. That's a point in the win column for me.

In *The Sun Also Rises* (1926), Hemingway travels to Pamplona during the Festival San Fermín, which is the home of the infamous running of the bulls. And so once again I followed in his footprints and ran with the bulls. It was exhilarating, arguably the best two minutes of my life—my honeymoon excluded.

Afterward, upon rereading that book, I realized with an even broader grin that Hemingway didn't actually run with the bulls either—he merely sat in a plaza, drinking wine all night. That's another point for me in the win column. For the record, he was likely another founding member of the bipolar club. For those keeping score, if Hemingway was considered a macho man, then I must be a macho macho man (apologies to the Village People).

I began my book project in 2017, making a killer debut with my first chapter, "I Killed Mom in Cold Ketchup." This was followed by "Climbing Kilimanjaro," "Jogging with the Bulls," "Wilt the Stilt," "The Anonymous Patriot," "Falling Down Mount Fuji," and "You're Only as Old as the Woman You Feel." Lastly, my instant classic, "Sex Toys," details an incident where I took a suitcase full of sex toys through security at Amsterdam Airport and was flagged as a potential terrorist for carrying plastic explosives. Apparently, the silicon in vibrators appears eerily similar to plastic explosives to a security scanner. Who knew? I won't reveal any more; you'll just have to buy the book *More Cowbell*. Soon to be a series streaming on either Netflix or Amazon—depending on who seals the deal first.

At MrClean Insane Asylum, writing in longhand, it takes me ten hours to finish my next masterpiece, "Area 51," breaking only for four double mochas. Here is an excerpt from this four-thousand-word chapter:

AREA 51

We're in Vegas and the guy on stage is killing it. "Speaking of Lovely Wife, she once brought me up on charges . . . assault with a dead weapon." Then it hits me, I WAS that guy. More on that later.

In 2011, my daughter had just graduated from high school. She cohosted a graduation party with a couple of her friends, and things got out of control towards the end. The large tent, which was used as the focal point, was collapsing. Chaos ensued with people scattering everywhere. We soon figured out that the main pole supporting the tent had snapped in two. One quick thinker ran for a broom stick, actually two, and I ran to get duct tape from my car. With several people supporting the top part of the pole, preventing the tent from collapsing entirely, we managed to "splint" the pole using the broomsticks and the duct tape. We couldn't believe it actually worked.

What the hell had happened? One of the kids yelled, "Ted did it." It turned out that one of the cohosts of the party had recently broken up with Ted, and he was clearly having a hard time with it. Ted's behavior towards his ex-girlfriend had become alarmingly erratic and dangerously intimidating.

At that moment, to get her away from the potential danger, I concocted a somewhat plausible idea. How about the three of us—my daughter, her friend, and I—embark on a road trip under the pretext of testing some fake driver's licenses? Naturally, if you're headed off to college where the drinking age is twenty-one, you're going to need a fake ID. First, we needed to acquire some state-of-the-art counterfeit driver's licenses. A quick Google search for "Which counterfeit state driver's licenses are the least likely to be detected?" Answer: California, Texas, Ohio, Rhode Island, and Connecticut. We opted for Rhode Island, being pretty sure that not many people had ever been to Rhode Island let alone seen a driver's license from there. So, who makes the best counterfeit IDs? China, of course. However, even in China quality doesn't come cheap.

Modern driver's licenses incorporate significant technology, such as holograms and laser perforations. It took $250 each to do the trick. However, it actually seemed like a bargain, because it was rumored that the Chinese factory we used manufactured the actual licenses for Rhode Island. The workers would work a late shift to make a little extra money on the side. The fakes would be real. One week later we had the goods.

Vegas is the gold standard for testing fake IDs. The casinos boast top-notch security, staff in well-pressed outfits, with earpieces, and they operate under strict regulations. It was clear that we had to do our test drive there: "If you can fake it there, you can fake it anywhere." At this point my running partner, Barry, overheard our plans and chimed in with a grin, "You know, there's an epic race outside Las Vegas in the middle of August? I'll look into it."

Before our big Vegas test, we needed a place to hone our skills. Even Broadway's best shows fine-tune their acts in other cities before their Big Apple debut. LA seemed like the perfect rehearsal stage as well as a fun adventure. As I was making reservations for the trip, Lovely Wife interjected, "This whole thing is nuts," and decided to join us to ensure the proverbial wheels didn't fall off the party bus.

We touched down in LAX and made our way to our five-star accommodation, the Fairmont Miramar in Santa Monica. We checked out the area, visited Muscle Beach, and the Santa Monica Pier. Back at the hotel, the girls put on their best "we're of legal age" outfit, and we headed for the Third Street Promenade. We were on the lookout for either a Chinese or Mexican restaurant, preferably both. The girls' research indicated that these two genres were more lenient when checking IDs, especially Chinese restaurants. At this point, I should mention that my daughter had just turned eighteen but looked more like fourteen. Her mother and I were thinking, *No way* they'd get in.

Right away we spotted a Chinese restaurant. Lovely Wife and I hung back. No one was stationed at the entrance, so the girls made a beeline for the bar. A minute ticked by, then another, and we began to think, Oh, no, it worked, they made it. Eventually, they walked out with big smiles on their faces and high-fived us. "No problem—they took the IDs at the bar and just handed them back," they reported, adding, "and we may have had a couple of drinks." I'm pretty sure that wasn't in the original script. On to Mexico.

Serendipitously, we didn't have far to go to as there was a Mexican restaurant right across the street. A guy in a sombrero was positioned outside the door, checking IDs. Since my daughter's friend appeared older, they decided she would take the lead. The girls approached with practiced confidence. Her friend chatted him up, and handed over her ID. He glanced at it, stepped aside, and let her in; my daughter followed in her wake. Once inside, the girls may or may not have had a margarita or two, they whispered something about the second round being "on the house."

The first act was a surprising success. We headed back to the Fairmont Hotel so the girls could sleep it off before our VEGAS opening. We Ubered back to LAX and found ourselves in a lengthy security line. A security guard informed us that Fridays were always like this. "The girls flock to Vegas for the weekend." Hmmm. What, exactly, did he mean by that rather cryptic comment? I quickly scanned the line, something seemed a little off. What was it? I'm supposed to be someone who can connect the dots pretty well. After the third dot, it clicked. The line was overwhelmingly female: tall, predominantly blondes and redheads, and how should I say it . . . extremely well-endowed. No doubt, this explained the rumored plastic shortage in LA.

We cleared security and headed to the gate. As luck would have it, most of the girls from the security line were also at our gate. We began to board, and since there were four of us, I graciously volunteered to let Lovely Wife, daughter, and her friend sit together. I "squeezed" into the middle seat in the next row. I was flanked by two of the Barbie dolls. I thought it only polite to chat them up, introduce myself, and explain that I had never been to Vegas—did they have any suggestions for what to do? We were having a lively conversation when Lovely Wife popped her head over the seat to ask about when we would be arriving. She didn't appear pleased and asked me to meet her in the aisle. She scolded, "I don't know how you managed that, but you're grounded." She quickly switched seats with me.

It was a short flight, and we landed at McCarran International Airport around noon, grabbed our Avis rental, and headed to the hotel. Not just any hotel—we had two rooms at the Mandarin Hotel, another five stars. It was spectacular, with a neat, understated, Asian theme, high-quality finishes and unparalleled service. Lovely Wife's one deal-breaker requirement—NO casino. She detested casinos. Her view was that they were populated by retirees wasting their social security checks (she was right about that) or gambling addicts tossing away their life's savings (she was right about that too). It was indeed a stunning hotel. However, I could only wonder: How could a luxury hotel in Vegas survive without a casino? Wasn't gambling the only reason you came to Vegas? Unsurprisingly, the hotel folded a few years later.

We rested up, and the girls, sans Lovely Wife, tried out their outfits and scoped out the places they would later visit that night. I couldn't help but notice their outfits were a bit too reminiscent of the ladies on the plane, but with shorter skirts. As they headed for the door, they shouted, "Find a comedy or magic act. We've heard they're good here. We'd like to see one." After some quick Googling, I found the perfect act, Mac King.

Penn and Teller described him as "The greatest comedy magician alive today, and maybe who ever lived. Mac King is a god." While I suspected that Penn and Teller might be getting a cut, I booked tickets anyway. Lovely Wife chose to sit this one out.

I met up with my friend Barry, who was also staying at the Mandarin. He was solo; his wife had zero interest in this endeavor and opted to stay home with their dog. Now, why was Barry in Vegas? Because I'm a bit ADHD, I like to do more than one thing at a time. When I mentioned my Vegas trip, he inquired about the dates. I told him August 12 through August 15. He smiled and asked, "You know what's on August 13th, right?" He knew I didn't have a clue. "It's the ET Full Moon race. They run a half-marathon straight through Area 51, at midnight. The best part, you run over a mountain." My immediate response, "Hell, yes, I'm in. See you in Vegas."

I tried to entice Barry to join us for Mac King's performance, but he declined, explaining, "The race is tonight. I need to rest up; it's going to be a long day and night." Knowing he liked to gamble, I was pretty sure that would be his version of resting. Later, he confessed that he had visited one of the sketchier casinos on the Strip downtown, lured by a low minimum, complementary drinks, and . . . TOPLESS waitresses. He said the $100 he parted with was the best investment he'd ever made. By this time, the girls had returned from their reconnaissance of the local clubs, and we headed for the 3:00 p.m. show at Harrah's, where Mac had played ten shows a week for the past eleven years.

The usher looked at our tickets and lead us to our seats, front row center aisle. The tickets were only $35 each—I didn't expect to get the FRONT ROW. I couldn't recall ever having front row seats for anything, except maybe an orca whale show at SeaWorld, where the front row got soaked. I asked the usher what made us so special. He indicated that we were the only ones who actually paid for our tickets, everyone else was comped, as in free tickets, by their hotels.

That's when the fun began. Mac took the stage and started by saying that his watch was broken and asked if anyone had the correct time. He emphasized that he liked to start his shows punctually. Well, I always know the exact time. I had two devices on me that were synced to the atomic clock located in Boulder, Colorado. Using the oscillation of the cesium 133 atom, they were accurate to one second every three hundred million years. I called out, "3:00:01—you're one second late." Everyone laughed. Mac responded, "Please join me on the stage." He then asked me for my name.

I pondered for a moment, then thought, Let's have some fun with my name. I've always admired how William James Adams Jr., of the Black Eyed Peas, ingeniously morphed his name, William, into will.i.am. So, I went for it, "Well, Mac, I am b.ill, and you don't want to be ill, do you?" Mac shook his head, laughed, and continued, "What brings you to Vegas?" I replied, "There's a full moon tonight, and they're hosting a half-marathon in the desert. "Area 51?" he asks. "Exactly, hence the name 'The ET Full Moon Half Marathon,'" I confirm. "Is your wife with you?" he pressed. "She's in Vegas, but not here." Mac asked, "Is she going to watch?" "No, she thinks it's stupid. Now, speaking of my Lovely Wife, she once brought me up on charges." Mac deadpans, "What charges?" I smirk. "Assault with a 'dead' weapon." Which is how this story begins. Mac stared at me in bemusement and said, "The stage is yours," then stepped aside.

I then elaborated, "Why am I here in Vegas? I got sucked into it by my friend Barry. We have a history of doing impulsive things together. This one seemed to fit the 'b.ill' (pun intended). We also like a challenge, particularly those that a sane person would think crazy. This race is grueling. Beginning at five thousand feet of elevation, the first six miles are up a relentless steep incline, ascending fifteen hundred feet into progressively thinner air. At the summit, I hope to be abducted by female aliens, whisked away to their spaceship, and forced to father a super species destined to rule the known universe."

Mac exclaimed, "You can't be serious!" I explained, "Well, at least that's the story I'm going to share with Lovely Wife when I stroll back into the hotel at 5:30 a.m. with a hooker on each arm, both wearing antennae." Glancing down to the front row, I noticed my daughter and her friend were unamused; they gave me the cut sign. I thanked my new pal, Mac, announced I'd be opening at Caesar's that upcoming Friday, and received a standing ovation. As I took my seat, despite the searing glare of the girls, I felt good—I had nailed it!

The remainder of the show was fantastic. A blend of illusions and comedic sketches. At the end of the show, Mac made his way to the back of the theatre and approached me, commenting, "You were a star." I asked him why he choose me to participate. He chuckled. "Your 'what time is it?' retort—3:00:01—made it impossible not to pick you. I'm looking for something different or quirky. You, my friend, ticked both boxes." Feeling pretty good about myself, I asked how my act ranked in his eleven-year tenure. Without hesitation he replied, "Number two?" Forget for the moment that I hate being a number two, his answer begged the question, "So, what was number one?"

It turned out that number one took place at a regional sales meeting for a very large tech company (think IBM). Mac didn't just perform his Vegas act; on one of his rare nights off, he moonlighted doing private events. That particular night, the head of sales, whom we'll call Mr. Slick, expressed his desire for his niece to be a part of the show. It was her sixteenth birthday, and he wanted it to be special for her.

Mac explained that he carefully selected audience members based on certain traits which he found significantly enhanced the magic experience. After all, he was the highest-rated magician in Vegas, so he must be doing something right. He respectfully declined. However, Mr. Slick insisted; his request was nonnegotiable—no niece, no pay. He pointed out his niece, seated in the front row, aisle seat.

Mac started with his usual opener: "Does anyone have the time?" That act went smoothly. For the next act he opted to pick the niece, deciding to get it out of the way. However, he didn't quite realize what he was about to do. He posed the question, "Does anyone have a birthday today?" A bubbly blonde in the front row excitedly raised her hand. Mac invited her onstage, and she rushed to join him. Forgetting she was only sixteen, he asked his usual second remark: "Pick a card or take off your clothes."

In a matter of seconds, the niece stood front and center, butt naked, looking like a goddess. We're talking Botticelli's *Venus* gorgeous. He finally snapped out of his daze and realized that his career was finished—completely done. He glanced at Mr. Slick, who shook his head and indicated a bullet to the head. What did he do next? The show had to go on.

The niece picked a card, Mac guessed it correctly, and he proceeded with the remaining acts.

At the end of the show, Mr. Slick walked over and asked Mac, “How do you think that went?” Mac began mumbling, but Mr. Slick interrupted, “Actually, it went really well, better than well—perfectly.” Mac thought, “What the fuck?” “Mac, you see, she isn’t my niece. That’s a stripper I hired for the night.”

The End

I’m finished, in every sense of the word. I realize that I’ve not only missed dinner, but also visiting hour. Jonah saved me some turkey, which I swallow in one gulp. I vaguely recall Lovely Wife mentioning she wouldn’t be coming tonight, allowing me to binge write. Head on pillow, eyes close, and I’m out.

CHAPTER 16

"HAVE YOU EVER BEEN MORE INTERESTED IN SEX THAN USUAL?"

DAY 14: MONDAY, AUGUST 13

For one last time, Jason calls in to say it's bathroom time. I step into the hallway, grab the towel, and head in. Today will be my last full day, and I'm planning on doing the Full Monty: bathroom routine, breakfast, movie, lunch, the walkabout, arts and crafts, a sit-down with Chief and Joey after their ECT, line up for dinner where I'll bid everyone . . . adieu, meet with Lovely Wife, and almost forgot, meet with Kerin's moms. Then back to the room to pack, talk with Jonah a bit, and finally, hit the sack.

Jonah and I head to breakfast and see Kerin sitting alone, a stark reminder that today is ECT day for Chief and Joey. I grab some scrambled eggs, and, halfway back to the table, I remember that I forgot the ketchup packet—the ones you can't easily open. And when you do, the ketchup often squirts out in a thin stream, which can travel several yards. Yeah, you read that right: I have ketchup on my eggs. Go ahead, judge me if you must, but that's how I like 'em.

I head back to my room to get an update on how things are going with the balls and cradle. I recall that Paul has all the materials now. I call him for an update.

"The balls are in my workshop. They look unbelievable. I used my giant calipers to measure, like Zach instructed. Every ball, from every direction, is exactly eight inches, and the nickel coating reflects better than a mirror."

He goes on, "However, since the surface is convex, the reflection makes you look fatter, not always a good look. You can see both yourself and the entire area behind you. Each ball weighs just over eighty pounds."

I ask, "Can you pick them up?"

Paul responds, "It's tricky, but I came up with a solution. The balls are slippery with no good place to grab. They're also really heavy and awkward to lift. Rubber gloves make it manageable."

He spurts out, "Now for the cradle, I'm heading to the stainless-steel mill today to make sure our job gets pushed to the front of the line. Manufacturing stainless tubing is a complex process involving more than twenty steps. Hopefully, they already have what we need in stock. If so, I'll load it into my truck. I have some pull with the guy at the loading dock—he's in my book club." I like it, blue-collar guys with Ivy League brains, or in Paul's case, more like an MIT brain.

Time for the movie. Kerin has cued up *Casablanca*, which, along with *Midnight in Paris* and *Animal House*, is one of my three favorite films. It's where Bogart delivers the unforgettable line, "We'll always have Paris," a sentiment echoed countless times by lovers parting for the last time. Given this is the last film we'll see together, I can't resist a "We'll always have MrClean."

Time to get amped up with another mocha and then work on a project I'd thought of earlier in the day. I still have some paper and a contraband pen in my room, and I decide to sketch my *Newton's Balls* for Kerin, Jonah, Joey, and Chief. I've talked about the balls a lot, and I'd like them to be able to "see" what the world's largest well-hung balls actually look like. Kerin will get to view them in action in about six weeks, but I want them all to have a reminder of what you can achieve when you follow your dreams. Of course, I achieved both a magnificent set of balls and . . . a ticket to MrClean.

As I mentioned earlier, I was an engineering student for a little less than a year. I was good at the math part, but struggled with the practical part, which included drawing complex 3D renderings. I simply couldn't do it, so I dropped out of engineering and into math, which was easy for me, and economics, which used baby math, making it even easier.

However, I could draw a 3D cube. Within this cube, I'm able to sketch out a pretty decent representation of how I imagine *Newton's Balls*.

Checking the time, I realize I'm running late for lunch.

However, the server gives a smile and says, "Last day. I set aside the turkey for you."

She piles on a double portion of the good stuff, earning a thumbs-up from me. I then make my way to the "popular table" with Jonah and Kerin in tow. Chief and Joey's usual seats are vacant, our version of the missing man formation.

We discuss our plans. Jonah is taking a semester off from Brandeis. Kerin will have three weeks in the facility in Tennessee. It turns out it is more like a halfway house than outpatient care. She is also going to practice for her big New York City debut at my art event.

She adds, "I forgot to mention, I still haven't told my moms about the show yet. That's your job tonight."

I exclaim, "Oy vey!"

Jonah laughs. "I didn't know you spoke Yiddish."

I affectionately retort, "I know a bit of vocabulary. 'Dr. Ratched is a schmuck,' for instance."

We all laugh.

Realistically, the relapse rate for mental "differences" is well above 50 percent. Chief and Joey aren't sure of their plans. I fear that their treatments might make it difficult for them to reenter society, so they are candidates, but Kerin and Jonah are as well. And how about me?

I keep thinking about MY post-release treatment. Nobody has provided me with the details, just that it will be two weeks of outpatient care at MrClean. The good news is that I'll have my Tesla. The bad news is that I don't know how to drive it, which I'll need for the daily thirty-mile roundtrip to MrClean. Worse yet, I'll be driving under the influence of my haze-inducing meds. On top of that, I'll need to carve out time for my art show preparation. Fortunately, I can stretch out my week, since, unlike doctors, I don't take weekends off. However, I do have to be careful since I earned my way into MrClean by stretching my days and weeks beyond the breaking point.

At 12:20 p.m., I head to my room and find my social worker, Debbie, from the catacombs, waiting. She gestures me to enter a phone booth–sized office I hadn't noticed before, where I am to take my neuropsych tests. The first one is the Mood Disorder Questionnaire, a thirteen-question test to determine if one is bipolar, or, more specifically, manic, which is all you need to earn a Bipolar I diagnosis.

Among the thirteen questions are "Have you ever felt much more confident than usual?" and "Have you ever shouted at someone whom you deem to be stupid?" My favorite is "Have you ever been more interested in sex than usual?" I answer the sex question honestly: "No." The reason being, I have always been interested in sex, 24/7/365, and on leap years, 24/7/366. So, it would be impossible for me to be more interested in sex than usual. Debbie told me I scored a 12/13, indicating I'm highly manic. I'm sure I know which question I missed.

The second, the Patient Health Questionnaire (PHQ-9), is a nine-question assessment used to determine if one suffers from depression, and, if so, its severity. A zero score suggests absolutely no signs of depression, while a score of nine indicates you're acutely depressed. I'm amused by the lack of subtlety of these questions:

"Over the past two weeks have you been bothered by feeling down, depressed, or hopeless?"

"Have you been feeling bad about yourself, or that you're a failure, or have let yourself or your family down?"

And the best for last, number nine: "Have you ever had thoughts that you would be better off dead or hurting yourself in some way?"

Where to begin with this test. First, my score: ZERO. It's always zero, no matter how many times they test me, and they test me a lot. Since my results are so consistent on the PHQ-9 test, they often follow up with a malingering test, meant to determine if you're lying about your answers. It's got a long title, the Minnesota Multiphasic Personality Inventory. They measure the consistency of your answers by presenting questions with minor variations and by rephrasing certain queries from "have you ever" to "have you never," for instance. The under(lying) theory suggests that nobody is perfectly consistent, and that even an honest test taker is expected to make a certain number of mistakes.

If you are totally consistent, and achieve the highest score for malingering, then they infer you must be manipulating the test. Hell, I figure they manipulate us by setting this trap, so why not play their game? By being too consistent in telling the truth, they assume I lie. The irony is that the only time I actually contemplate ending my life is after they've asked me variations of "Have you ever thought of ending your life?" a dozen or more times.

Now for the serious part. We know that thinking about something makes it more likely to occur. The psychiatric profession is deeply concerned about mentally ill individuals committing suicide. They frequently discuss suicidal ideation, constantly inquiring, "Do you have suicidal thoughts?" Well, here's the thing: The more you ask that question, the more people will have those thoughts. This CAN lead to increased suicidal ideation, resulting in more suicides. It becomes a self-fulfilling prophecy. Particularly disturbing is the copycat suicide, or suicide contagion.

The first documented case in 1774 was eventually coined the Werther Effect. Werther, the lead character in Goethe's book, *The Sorrows of Young Werther*, lost his true love to another. He shot himself in the head, and not unsurprisingly, died. He was wearing yellow pants and a blue jacket. Soon after the book was published, it was reported that numerous young men suffering from unrequited love killed themselves by self-inflicted gunshot wounds while wearing yellow pants and a blue jacket.

Starting in the 1970s, the medical community in the US became increasingly aware of the Werther Effect. Particularly troubling was a pattern of subsequent suicides occurring within close proximity to the original suicide. The prevailing theory was that the publicity around the initial suicide was causing this contagion. This phenomenon is now so widely accepted that responsible newspapers typically avoid publishing the cause of death in suicide cases, just something generic like, "The family requests privacy during this difficult time."

Perhaps the most notable case of copycat suicides involved the death of universally worshipped sex goddess Marilyn Monroe. It was reported at the time that in August 1962, over two hundred suicides by young females were attributable to Marilyn's death by barbiturate overdose.

Now, for perhaps the most perplexing fact about suicide. Let me start with a quiz. Which profession has the highest suicide rate?

a. Dentists
b. Police Officers
c. Veterinarians
d. Financial Services Professionals
e. None of the above

Obviously, the answer must be A) Dentists. Their job requires them to inflict pain on their patients, and that must take a toll on their soul. The most famous dental torture scene is in the movie *Marathon Man*, 1976. I wouldn't recommend watching it, as you might never go to the dentist again, which would condemn you to a toothless old age. Sir Laurence Olivier plays a Nazi war criminal, Dr. Christian Szell, who has successfully stolen and concealed a massive stash of diamonds from Auschwitz prisoners, who subsequently perished.

Dustin Hoffman plays "Babe" Levy, the brother of a secret government agent working for the United States, whose mission is to track down Szell. A huge hoard of diamonds is stashed in New York. Szell's goal is to bring the diamonds back to South America, where he is residing. He kills Babe Levy's brother and, incorrectly believing that Babe knows the location of the diamonds, takes him to the Reservoir in Central Park. To extract the information, he tortures Babe by drilling through one of his live teeth. I am still haunted by Babe's agonized screaming every time I'm in the dentist's chair. Babe escapes using his prowess as a marathon runner.

Back to the test: Surprisingly the answer is not A) Dentists, B) Police officers, C) Veterinarians, or D) Financial Services Professionals. The correct answer is E) none of the above. The actual answer is medical doctors, and the subspecialty within medicine with the highest suicide rate is psychiatrists!

The job of a psychiatrist, as it currently stands, is almost impossible. It is the perfect storm. A patient presents with some form of mental health issue. The psychiatrist diagnoses it, often asking repeatedly if the patient has had suicidal thoughts. The recommended treatment is prescribed, which most of the time doesn't work. Then another med is tried, which also fails. The patient then switches to a new doctor, who prescribes a different med, which likewise doesn't work, and so on.

These patients contemplate suicide, and some actually go through with it. Over ten years, even the best psychiatrist will have more of these cases than anyone should. So, what does the doctor think about a lot? Suicide, probably thousands of times—more than any of their patients do. And thinking is ideation. Suicidal "ideation" is the most common precursor to suicide, hence the not-so-surprising result.

Back to me. Debbie then announces my fate: two weeks in the outpatient ward at MrClean. Not a surprise since Jason has already given me a heads-up. I decide to have some fun with it.

"So, Dr. Ratched sent you as the sacrificial lamb?" I suggest.

She knows I have an important show at the end of October and will not appreciate this news. I need to be home, without this added stress, focusing on my task ahead. I will likely be disruptive to everyone else at outpatient. Not to mention, I'll be a menace to both cars and pedestrians as I drive roundtrip in my new Tesla, which I have no clue how to operate.

I add, "You can tell Dr. Ratched that I appreciate her help and that one day she'll be one of the main characters in my book. I'll call her . . . Dr. Ratched. On second thought, keep that one between us."

I head straight to the signup board for the outing. As has become customary lately, someone has penciled me into the coveted number one spot. I return to the room to get Jonah and meet Kerin on the way. I'm feeling a bit nostalgic as we navigate the subterranean rabbit warren to reach the door to the gym one last time. Once there, my fellow wardmates start doing "exercises." One is touching, not their toes, but their knees. Another is doing "jumping jacks," only without the jumping. You could generously call them arm raises. Several of them are just standing, shaking their arms. Finally, I get it: they are warming up for the circular ball pass. Jonah takes charge, saying, "All right, everyone. Line up in a circle."

Surprisingly, they do. With Kerin to my left and Jonah to my right, I hand the ball to Kerin, who hands it to the person to her left. This continues, and, to my surprise, it's going quite well. Eventually, the ball makes it to Jonah, who hands it to me.

Rather than disbanding, the group stays put as Jonah declares, "The Captain leaves tomorrow. Let's do one more round for him."

And so it goes. I end up with the ball once again, and as the group cheers, I tell Jonah and Kerin, "You guys are now the cocaptains of Circle Pass."

They smile and toss the ball to Jason, who is also laughing. We line up and open the door to the bright and beautiful outdoors.

The sunlight instantly reminds me of one of the things I've detested most about MrClean. You now know the punchline of my joke, no joke, "What's the difference between being in solitary at the most secure prison in the world and me being placed in the secure section of the ward at MrClean?" But humor me. I'm told it's good therapy to talk these things out. The worst of the worst felons are held at the most secure prison in the world, called a "supermax," more formally known as a super-maximum-security prison.

For those of you who have never had the pleasure of staying at a supermax prison, or visiting a loved one there, allow me to elucidate. These prisons are considered impossible to escape from. They've got all the cool electronic gear seen in the Tom Cruise *Mission Impossible* movies, and more: iris scan door locks, motion detectors, lasers, high-def cameras, infrared cameras, sonar, and good old-fashioned boots on the ground.

Alcatraz was the first and remains the most infamous one. However, the ADX Florence Supermax Prison in Colorado has now superseded it. Current "guests" include Dzhokhar Tsarnaev, a.k.a. the Boston Marathon Bomber, who killed three people and wounded 260 during the 117th running of the race in 2013; Timothy McVeigh, a.k.a. the Oklahoma Bomber, who killed 168 people, and my personal favorite, Joaquín Guzmán, a.k.a. El Chapo, the most powerful drug lord in the world, who admits to being responsible for killing more than two thousand people.

Back to the question I posed earlier, "What's the difference between being in solitary at the most secure prison in the world and me being placed in the secure section of the ward at MrClean?"

The answer is—you guessed it—all of the worst of the worst are allowed one hour outside each day. Me? Zilch. At least until I blew the whistle. It seems they considered me a bigger threat to society than all of that pure evil put together. They justified it by claiming I was an existential threat to myself—my own worst enemy, and not only likely to harm myself, but maybe do them harm. So, they took away some of the most powerful reasons for me to live, sunlight and fresh air. Also, remember that I'm clinically claustrophobic. Not a good thing when you are locked up. Nice going. Once again, I'll suggest a little empathy training, MrClean psychiatrists. Lock yourselves up in a room 24/7, not allowed to leave, and see how it makes you feel. Better or worse?

Now on to a much more pleasant thought. I am walking with two new friends I met here, Kerin and Jonah, on a beautiful day. Even though they are forty-five years younger than me, we have formed an unlikely bond and developed a symbiotic relationship whereby we are all better off for knowing each other. We are powerful medicine, and once again, no cost and no side effects. I'm not sure that was part of MrClean's plan.

We decide to exchange our contact information, which is strictly forbidden, making it all the more appealing. However, if brought up on charges, any jury would likely rule "innocent by reason of insanity," using MrClean's own diagnosis.

Jason, who is usually quite taciturn, starts talking. He admits that our group has solidified a feeling he has had for a while.

"Nursing, in general, is a very stressful job. However, patients admitted into a regular hospital usually have an issue that can be both diagnosed and successfully treated. At MrClean, the patients are at the last stop of the mental health train. Nothing else has helped them, so they use very aggressive treatments here. The most aggressive treatment is ECT, and it's performed more here than any other mental institution. One hundred thousand patients receive ECT treatments nationwide—every year. Their biggest fear is that patients will take their own lives."

At this point, I speak the unspeakable: "Perhaps some of the patients are better off not having to suffer a lifetime of pain that can't be cured. Maybe it's time to let Sisyphus stop pushing the stone."

He gives a soft nod with a subtle grimace. Jason goes on to say that I wasn't wrong when I noticed that the nurses spend more time covering the collective asses of the hospital than on patient care. "Lawsuits are considered enemy number one, and self-harm often leads to one."

Again, I interject, "And the hired lawyers make enough money to buy their Nantucket summer homes."

He ends by saying, "I'm thinking of switching professions altogether."

Many of his colleagues have gone to the "other side"—some refer to it as the "dark side." Working for a healthcare company as a sales rep, Jason would be a good fit; he knows the lingo and understands the customers' needs.

He reveals, "I've been thinking about this for a while, and the last two weeks have solidified my decision. I've really enjoyed your complete disdain for management, and that's why I may have helped you a bit."

With a broad smile, he gives me a high five.

I'm taken slightly off guard, but not really surprised when I hear his admission.

He continues, "Your party has gone viral, not only within the MrClean community but well beyond."

At this point, we're back to the flower garden, meander through the labyrinth, and enter the ward. Chief and Joey are waiting for us in the activity room with expressionless faces.

I ask them to wait a minute while I get my meds, a mocha—no surprise to any of you paying attention.

As I sit down, Chief speaks up, "It's not getting any better, even worse now that I know what comes afterward. But I'll hang in there as long as you think it will help—but it's not easy."

Joey adds, "It was the worst experience of my life, and I feel like shit."

For the umpteenth time I realize I have no choice but to reassure them. However, at this point, I'm really starting to feel like shit myself. I'm an alchemist trying to turn lead into gold, only I have to turn a lie into a truth. In my defense, I'm in good company here. I have the big three backing me up: the placebo effect, the self-fulfilling prophecy, and the not yet mentioned reality distortion field, or RDF.

"So, what the hell is RDF?" you might ask. It is an expression first used to describe Apple's Steve Jobs's loose relationship with the truth. In 1981, Bud Tribble, an Apple employee, first coined the term. It was borrowed from a 1966 *Star Trek* episode, "The Menagerie," in which aliens could create their own reality through mental willpower. Tribble used it to describe Jobs's ability to bend reality to his advantage. Critics of Jobs said he was lying, but the engineers at Apple reluctantly suggested otherwise. He would make a statement such as, "I will reduce the boot up time of the Macintosh by ten seconds."

Everybody knew this was unachievable, including the engineer in charge of the project, Barry Kenyon.

Jobs asked him, "Could you do it if it saved someone's life?"

Kenyon replied, "Yes."

Jobs then illustrated on a whiteboard how saving ten seconds each for five million users would result in one hundred human lifetimes saved per year. Two weeks later, Kenyon had rewritten the code and shaved off—wait for it—twenty-eight seconds from the boot-up time. That's THREE HUNDRED human lifetimes per year.

Elon Musk, same story. He declared that he was going to alter the trajectory of the automobile industry, one dominated by the Big Three: Toyota, Volkswagen, and Hyundai. Yep, you read that right—not GM, Ford, and Chrysler—but that's a topic for yet another book. And how was he going to do it? Electric vehicles (EVs).

The critics smugly proclaimed that the batteries would not allow cars an adequate range, and the charging stations would be too slow—not to mention, not enough of them. One more of Elon's wild claims was that the cars would be fully self-driving (FSD). How did he do? The batteries had a great range of over three hundred miles, and there were plenty of fast-charging stations, more than forty thousand. Not so good on the FSD, though—to avoid using a couple of George Carlin's works, let's just say less than stellar.

Elon also did the same with rockets. In what will be a surprise to many, he actually cofounded SpaceX before becoming involved with Tesla. The "experts" proclaimed, "It's impossible to reuse a rocket, let alone to re-land one." However, Elon found a way. What was the common link between Jobs and Musk? They had delusions of grandeur that turned into reality through sheer will and charisma. They were modern-day Jesuses and . . . as bipolar as you can get.

That's all a roundabout way of saying, "I can justify my lie and do Dr. Norman Vincent Peale proud."

I tell Chief and Joey, "It will work."

They both look a little less zombie-like. The follow-up discussion is a bit more difficult. Would ECT affect Chief's wrestling or Joey's world-class gaming skills?

I'm not really sure, so I tell them, "First things first. Let's get your heads feeling better, and then you can focus on regaining your other talents."

Now, let's take a serious detour, and in some cases a deadly serious detour—a deeper dive into what we think we know about electroconvulsive shock therapy and its predecessor, the lobotomy. I now have a better idea of what Chief and Joey should expect with respect to how ECT might affect their world-class wrestling and video game performance. A 2010 meta-analysis of eighty-four studies, published in *Biological Psychiatry* suggests that Chief and Joey are most likely screwed. Among other effects, processing speed can be significantly diminished, both short term and long term.

Wrestling requires split-second decisions to counter your opponent's moves, and even worse, milliseconds of delay in gaming takes you from winning the race to an also-ran. Most discouraging, research suggests that as many as 50 percent of ECT patients relapse. In fact, severely depressed people, due to their low energy and motivation, often lack the ability to act on their suicidal ideations. However, ECT might actually give them enough energy to do so—think Ernest Hemingway.

To be fair, there are many published articles that purport to show that ECT is effective. However, these articles all share an interesting trait. In their footnotes, they reference other articles that reach the same conclusion, that ECT is the "gold standard." Yet most of these "other articles" are based on the same few articles. If one hundred articles cite the same article showing the efficacy of ECT, we don't have one hundred independent articles supporting the conclusion; we have just one. This mirrors the problem with social media: One wacko posts that voting machines are controlled by aliens, and thousands of wacko wannabes retweet it. What looks like an avalanche of support is merely one voice echoed over and over. Maybe one of the patients at MrClean started that one—alien conspiracy theories are popular here.

The fundamental problem is that the medical community does not fully understand what causes mental illness, or how to cure it. With ECT, they believe they have a treatment that helps treat a patient's "illness," or at least some of the symptoms. However, the degree of effectiveness is unclear, while the negative side effects are clear—side effects I have witnessed.

John Read's April 5, 2021, article in *Psychiatric Times* titled "ECT: Dangerous on Either Side of the Pond," concludes, "There is no evidence that ECT is better than placebo beyond the end of the treatment period, there is no evidence that it saves lives, and studies have found that it causes persistent or permanent memory loss in 12% to 55% of patients, with particularly high rates among women and older individuals."

I suppose it's time to drill down a bit on the lobotomy. It's a surgical procedure that severs the prefrontal cortex from the rest of the brain. Imagine drilling a hole in the front of someone's skull and using an ice pick to sever nerves. The prefrontal cortex controls personality, free will, and aspects of speech. After the treatment, many patients become complacent, even zombie-like.

In the movie *One Flew over the Cuckoo's Nest*, the lobotomy was the treatment that finally ended Jack Nicholson's reign as chief tormentor during his stay at Oregon State Hospital (OSH)—portrayed as an insane asylum. As mentioned earlier, Nicholson's character, Randle Patrick McMurphy, pretends to be mentally ill to avoid prison time for statutory rape. From the beginning of his incarceration, he is insubordinate and threatens the authority of Nurse Ratched, who is cold, controlling, heartless, cruel, maybe even evil.

Nurse Ratched is all-powerful within OSH and does as she pleases, especially to those who displease her. From the beginning, she knows McMurphy will be a problem. She gives him a round of electroconvulsive shock treatment, but much to her chagrin, it has no effect. He still has enough wherewithal to make her life unbearable. He one-ups me in the party category by sneaking in two prostitutes, along with plenty of alcohol, and they really "dance" the night away.

But wait, there's more. McMurphy's close patient friend Billy Bibbit takes his own life, after being driven to despair when Nurse Ratched threatens to disclose to his mother that he had sex with one of the prostitutes at the party. McMurphy is so enraged that he tries to strangle Nurse Ratched.

At this point, she retaliates by authorizing the thermonuclear option, a lobotomy. Once more, it is considered the "gold standard" at the time for controlling the uncontrollable.

Anticipating this potential outcome, McMurphy has previously arranged with his ally, Chief, that he doesn't want to live in a lobotomized state. The film ends with Chief mercifully suffocating McMurphy to end his suffering. Chief then makes a daring escape by hurling a huge desk through a window and running into the woods. Thus, Chief becomes the symbolic "one" who "flew over the cuckoo's nest."

The history of lobotomy goes back to Swiss physician Gottlieb Burckhardt, who first performed the procedure in 1888. He had an epiphany: that it might subdue unruly patients. His method involved using a manual hand drill, like the ones used in high school workshop classes, to shred the prefrontal cortex. However, after six procedures with catastrophic outcomes, his medical peers intervened, deeming it torture and prohibiting him from performing any more.

António Egas Moniz, a Portuguese neurologist, picked up the drill again in 1935. He coined the term "lobotomy," derived from the Greek words *lobo*, meaning lobe, and *tome*, to cut. For his pioneering work, he won the Nobel Prize in Medicine in 1949. Fittingly, that prize was made possible by Alfred Nobel, who established and funded the Nobel prizes in 1901. Ironically, Nobel made his fortune by inventing dynamite, which the military used at the time to kill more efficiently.

The breakthrough with the lobotomy came in 1945, when Walter Freeman and James Watts used a spatula, after drilling through the skull, to sever the prefrontal cortex more efficiently, allowing for more procedures to be performed. Then—wait for it—they actually did use an ice pick, inserted up the patient's nose, rotated it a few times, and in ten minutes, everything was done.

Walter Freeman became the go-to guy, performing as many as thirty-five hundred lobotomies during his ignominious career. The "golden years" for this "gold standard" procedure spanned from 1949 to 1952, with about fifty thousand lobotomies performed.

Rosemary Kennedy, the first daughter of Joseph P. Kennedy and sister of President John F. Kennedy, was one of the most renowned recipients of a lobotomy. Joe Sr. had an interesting past, reportedly making a fortune as a bootlegger during prohibition, and then buying a Hollywood studio to fraternize with numerous starlets.

Rosemary became physically and intellectually disabled due to oxygen deprivation at birth. Her situation became more perilous when, in 1938, she stumbled during a curtsy to Queen Elizabeth. Her father was morbidly embarrassed. Shortly thereafter, he placed her in a nunnery where she euphemistically "acted out" with boys, a further embarrassment for a good Catholic family.

Joe Sr.'s ultimate ambition was to see one of his sons become president. The oldest son, Joe Jr., was the primary candidate. He was smart, good-looking, and, of course, appealed to the ladies. In 1941, to protect the family from further disgrace and smooth the path to the White House for both Joe Jr. and himself, Joe Sr. authorized a relatively new procedure—a lobotomy—for Rosemary.

Tragically, the procedure further reduced her intellectual capacity to that of a two-year old. Joe Sr. hid the news from his family. More tragedy struck when Joe Sr.'s plans were derailed in 1944, when Joe Jr. died during a World War II bombing mission. Rather than give up on his dream, Joe Sr. slotted son number two into position, despite his reputation as a womanizer.

Back to the story. I once again reassure Chief and Joey that it's going to be okay. Once again, I know it's bullshit, but they can't know it's bullshit. We sit in silence, and they seem somewhat comforted. After about an hour, I walk them back to their respective rooms, and we agree to meet in the cafeteria tonight for my "last supper." I continue to feel frustrated and helpless. They will get their treatments, they will most likely suffer bad side effects, and the only hope of some positive result is the placebo effect—to tell them it will help.

I leave Chief and Joey with the one positive thing about their ECT treatments I can think of: "Chief, you are done with your treatments, and, Joey, you are halfway through."

I head back to the room.

Once again, the woman behind the counter hands me a plate with the turkey she's reserved for me. I thank her; she nods. As I pivot to our table, I realize that Jonah intentionally delayed us—everyone is standing. Most are holding pie plates with messages: Jason the nurse writes, "Run, Captain, run," Slugger says, "Stay in touch," Chief displays, "Let's rumble," Joey holds up, "You are my avatar," and there are a few more.

I look over to Kerin; she smiles and holds up a plate that reads, "I will miss you." She flips it over to reveal: "Unicorn." Finally, Jonah holds up a plate that says, "Best Roommate Ever." With a few tears rolling down my cheeks, I give a double thumbs-up and sit down.

Joey, Kerin, Jonah, and Chief all join me.

As we settle in, Kerin inquires, "You know, we don't know much about you. What's YOUR story?"

I'm caught off guard, but it's a fair question.

I respond, "The short answer is that you'll have to read my book."

"What book?" Jonah asks somewhat incredulously.

I give them a brief primer on my spiritual awakening on Mount Fuji and the promise I made to improve humanity in some significant way.

"Who better than me to tell the world how insane the treatment of the insane can be, and how we need to change it? The best part?

You guys will be the main characters, along with Lovely Wife, of course." I summarize the book's message with, "Where there is joy, there is life."

Time to get back to my room, prepare my high-test mocha, and await Kerin's moms.

At exactly 7:00 p.m., Kerin swings by and says, "Showtime."

I give her a thumbs-up and head out to the greeting area. Two smiling women greet me with a contraband hug. Kerin introduces them as Jane and Ellen.

We head to the activity room and take our seats. After some chitchat, they express their gratitude for the support I've given Kerin and how she seems happier.

I tell them, "Kerin was the first one to show me kindness in this place. She told me, 'Don't worry, I'll help you get out of here,' and she was right. I'm out of here tomorrow."

Lovely Wife has reminded me that despite my frustration—and antics—I am getting out in near record time. Most are here for many weeks, even many months, while some never leave—alive.

Then the conversation turns more serious. They explain that one of the reasons Kerin is struggling with "issues" is that she is a perfectionist, particularly with her singing. They are worried that her performance at my upcoming show might put too much pressure on her and exacerbate her condition.

At this point, I ask Kerin for a few minutes alone with her parents. She nods and leaves the room.

Using my empathy training, I begin, "I hear your concerns, and they're absolutely valid. However, based on my observations, Kerin is an exceptionally talented singer. The positive reinforcement she could gain from the New York experience might be exactly what she needs to boost her self-esteem and give her a much-deserved sense of pride. Plus, she'll have the support of both of you accompanying her to the city, being there with her, and taking her to the event."

Fortunately, they buy it and agree to let Kerin sing. I bid them . . . adieu and give Kerin a thumbs-up as she rejoins her mothers.

She shouts, "YES!" in triumph.

As her moms depart, I notice Lovely Wife entering. I ask her how her day is going.

She grins slightly and says, "Still doing the 'fake it till you make it' empathy thing? I suppose it's better than no empathy."

Deciding to take this to the next level, I approach her, touch her arm in the safe zone—shoulder to elbow, as I have been trained to do—look into her eyes, and ask, "It seems like something may be bothering you. Would you like to talk about it?"

She pulls away, laughing, and retorts, "YOU are what's bothering me."

I reply, "Touché."

Lovely Wife then reminds me that I have a window between 11:00 a.m. and 1:00 p.m. tomorrow to pick up my Tesla, "or else they give it to the next person on the list." "Assholes," I say to myself.

She continues, "Also, Dr. Welby, your primary care physician, wants to see you as soon as you are released. You have an 8:00 a.m. appointment at MorAss General tomorrow. Most importantly, don't forget you start your two-week program tomorrow at MrClean's outpatient center, near the parking lot," she reminds me, as if I know where that is. "They will give you the details in your discharge papers."

She bids me . . . adieu.

Back in the room, I grab my room-temperature cup of high-test-coffee and a packet of Nestlé cocoa powder. I tell Jonah I'll be back in two minutes, then head to the cafeteria microwave to heat my mocha. I suppose you could call this a coffee break, which brings to mind one of Lovely Wife's favorite songs from the Broadway musical *How to Succeed in Business Without Really Trying*, one of the greatest tributes to the only drug that really seems to help me in Summer Camp: "Coffee Break."

If I can't take my coffee break
My coffee break, my coffee break . . . If I can't take my coffee
break, Something within me dies.

"Coffee Break,"* How to Succeed in Business, *1961

Upon returning to my room, I find Jonah engrossed in coding his digital art for his upcoming show at Brandeis.

He looks up and says, "I just found out I'm getting out the day after you. Thank God. I didn't want another roommate."

But, of course, he probably will have another roommate for his last day. There's a long line of people waiting to get in here. Unless you know someone with enough clout to move you to the front of the line, you'll probably have to go elsewhere.

Let me see: The idea of lining up for the cure brings to mind the French Revolution, specifically the infamous Reign of Terror. Back then, people with mental differences were labeled *dérangés*. They would be lined up to receive what was considered the "ultimate treatment," which not only cured their illness but also rid society of their disruptive behavior. This infallible treatment involved "offing" their heads, a method even more efficient than the lobotomy—the guillotine. It was perfected by Joseph-Ignace Guillotin in 1789. I had the privilege of visiting his home in Paris where he experimented using sheep in his courtyard; much to the dismay of his neighbors, the bleating turned into bleeding.

Perhaps the most renowned victim of the guillotine was "off with her head" Marie Antoinette, Queen of France, who actually did lose her head in 1793 along with tens of thousands of those of lower rank during the infamous Reign of Terror. This "gold standard" method was still used until September 10, 1977. On that date, Hamida Djandoubi, a Tunisian convicted of torture and murder, became the last person to be chopped. Interestingly, for a period, guillotining, lobotomies, and electroconvulsive shock treatment coexisted.

"Looks like I'm also in the outpatient program," Jonah says. "Two weeks, same as you. We'll overlap for most of it."

Strangely enough, Jonah seems excited about this, perhaps because we'll have more time together.

I offer Jonah a perfunctory "Sounds great" while concentrating on my packing. With my early departure, I worry that I'll have morning haze, so I must make sure everything is good to go now. Especially important to me are the ten cans of DawnMist Shave Cream I have stashed away.

One last item on my list: the brown PJs. I'm not entirely sure what I'll do with them, but I'm taking them anyway.

As I lie in bed, I ponder my time here.

A friend who visited me remarked, "You'll probably call this 'one of your greatest experiences ever.'"

He's not wrong. How many can claim they've been locked up in the country's premier insane asylum? And of those, how many stayed clear-headed enough to recount it accurately?

I'm "pumped up" and prepared to honor my vow made on Mount Fuji, to make a major contribution to humankind.

CHAPTER 17

"FREEDOM"

DAY 15: MONDAY, AUGUST 14

It's my last day, and I wake up at 5:00 a.m. I sit quietly in my bed, not wanting to disturb Jonah, who was up late working on his show. I begin formulating a mental checklist for my book's central theme and the multitude of examples that support my central assertion, "Shame on you—we can do much, much better than the status quo."

Checking the time, I head for the door. Yesterday, Jason mention that he'd work the early shift and would meet me by the exit door at 7:00 a.m.—my release time. I get there a little early and schedule an Uber with a pickup time of 7:15 a.m. to meet me at the main entrance. I'm a bit worried about navigating the labyrinth on my own for the first time. I have a terrible sense of direction, even on a good day.

Jason arrives exactly on time, holding yet another can of DawnMist Shave Cream.

He hands it to me with a grin, saying, "It's a gift from the staff. We all thought it was hysterical when we saw you hoarding these. Everyone signed it—well, everyone except—wait for it—Dr. Ratched."

I shake his hand, replying, "Thanks. Couldn't have done it without you."

He hands me the discharge papers.

His final words are, "You've made our wall of fame, which is not easy; your party sealed the deal."

Without a glance at the papers, I rip them in half and toss them into the trash can. Lovely Wife will no doubt have all the details—she never trusts me with important documents anyway.

Partway through the maze, I'm hopelessly lost, or to use my late brother's favorite word once again—*flummoxed.* There have been countless forks in the road. I recall the old Yogi Berra quip: "When you come to a fork in the road, take it." It's not so funny now. My strategy becomes take a right, then a left, right, left, right, left. I figure this way, I won't circle back to where I started.

Just then, I hit a dead end, with a closed door labeled "boiler room."

I'm thinking, *Give me a fucking break.* My next thought is that for some unknown reason, I haven't used as many George Carlin words in the last week or so. Well, no one's going to give a shit about that, and I retrace my steps using the modified left-right strategy and end up—predictably—right where I started. I see someone approaching and contemplate a virtually impossible task for those of us with an XY chromosome: asking for directions.

Before I can speak, the kind woman says, "You look lost. Need some help?" and jokingly adds, "You wouldn't be the first."

Gratefully, I reply, "Thank you so much."

I'm appreciative for the assistance, and much more importantly, I didn't have to ask for directions; my lifetime streak is intact.

"I have no sense of direction," I admit.

She asks, "Where are you headed?"

"To the front entrance. I'm being released."

She offers, "That's on my way. I'll take you there."

Of course, the last time I heard "That's on my way" was when the pervert molested me hitchhiking from the skating rink where I first held hands with Sweet Sue. However, this time I'm sure I'm safe. We reach the door, I open it and walk out, and the door shuts behind me as I flip a double bird to Summer Camp.

My Uber's waiting. The fare to MorAss General, $12.90. No surge pricing right now, perhaps a good omen. I arrive and head straight to Dr. Welby's office. The receptionist informs me that he's waiting, and before I can even enter the examination room, he appears.

He gives me a big hug and says, "You'll be fine. Outpatient won't be too bad, and after two weeks, you're good to go. How's your show coming along?"

"Still a long way to go before the end of October," I respond.

He offers, "Work with your psychiatrist on your meds. He thinks there's a better way to go than what you're on now."

I know he's referring to getting me off the mind-numbing shit they gave me at MrClean, but at least I avoided the ECT, and I take my leave.

I once again fire up my Uber app and set the destination for "Tesla Dealership Needham." Once inside, an overly enthusiastic Tesla advisor greets me from behind a tall desk. I inform him I'm here to pick up my Tesla. He confirms my identity, checks the computer, and heads out to retrieve my paperwork. He returns quickly with a large envelope, I sign one form, and he hands me two black key cards and escorts me to the car.

"Enjoy your vehicle," he says, with no further instructions. He indicates that the car virtually drives itself and leaves.

I get into the Tesla and Google "How to put the Tesla Model 3 into reverse," and then "drive," and I'm off. And then I stop. "Off to where?" I figure I'll start with Paul at the steel fabrication place and see how the balls are hanging. I Google "How to use the GPS in the Tesla Model 3?" then punch in the address, and I'm off for real this time.

As I merge onto Route 128 North, I notice traffic approaching from the left, so I floor it. My head jerks back, my hands lift off the wheel for a second, and I catch a glimpse of tiny specks in the rearview mirror that look like itty bitty cars.

I slow down and notice the speedometer on the big screen to my right reads 102. I'm not sure if that's kilometers per hour or miles per hour, so I look again and see it reads "102 miles per hour." I can't help but smile and exclaim, "Cool!" I'm liking the "preposterous" mode, for which I shelled out an extra 10K. It's worth every thousand.

I exit onto the Route 90 Eastbound and head to South Boston, where Smith & Son's Steel Works is located. Upon entering, the office manager, who knows me well by now, gestures toward Paul. I wander over and find the stainless-steel cradle looking fabulous and reflecting like a mirror. The balls are sitting next to the cradle, shrink-wrapped with clear protective film to preserve the mirror finish. The covering will remain on until the balls are hanging in GB's SoHo gallery, to ensure they don't get a single scratch.

Paul informs me that he and Zach have figured how to attach the balls to the wires and the wires to the cradle. He'll have the balls attached in a few days. I give him a hug and commend him for his most excellent work.

He thanks me for giving him the chance to work on what he calls his "favorite project ever, by far."

I mention I'm heading over to see Brad Tolman at his shop.

Paul laughs and remarks, "Good luck with that."

As I might have mentioned earlier, Brad has a reputation for being an eccentric curmudgeon, which is both well-deserved and likely why we get along so well.

Half a mile away, I pull into the parking lot of Tolman Manufacturing and Supply's and spot Brad's 1979 Toyota Camry, which proudly displays 315,000 miles on its odometer. Now, it's not for lack of bread, like the Grateful Dead. Brad owns his business and the land it sits on, with zero debt. The property, situated on the Bass River feeding into Boston Harbor, is contiguous with downtown Boston and the intersection of two major highways, Route 93 and Route 90, which the locals call the Mass Pike. Adjacent to his property is the world's largest Gillette manufacturing center. They produce more razor blades there than anyone else, anywhere. Gillette is always looking to expand and has likely offered Brad tens of millions for his lot.

Brad owns a fleet of exotic cars, with a vintage Mercedes being his favorite. He claims it's fast, but refuses to drag race my Tesla, "title for title"—a term we used in the 1960s where the winner would claim the title of the loser's car.

I shout, "BRAD!" at the loading dock, and he ambles out, resembling a vagrant more than a titan of gas.

He knows why I'm here and quips, "They should have kept you in the slammer. I've got my own work to do."

I laugh and retort, "I was only in the slammer because you're dragging out this project. How's it going?"

"Nowhere," he grunts. "I guess I have to get back to it."

I tell him, "I've got work release classes, but I'll be stopping by every morning at 6:00 a.m. to check on the progress. You're as excited about the *Rising Snowflakes* project as I am; you're just a cantankerous old man, but I've got your number."

"Okay," he concedes.

He walks me back to my car and asks, "So what can this thing do again?"

I tell him, "Zero to sixty in 3.1 seconds, with a top speed of 155."

He corrects me, "You can go faster than that. They limit the speed to 155 in the software. I can bypass that, and you can probably hit closer to 200."

I propose that once he finishes the project, I might let him have a go at it. I hop in the car, having left the door open since basic functions like opening the door, trunk, or glovebox are still eluding me, and head home.

I arrive home and park outside the garage, unable to open the garage door until I program the "HomeLink" feature of the car. Finally, I've solved the mystery of opening the car door from the inside and hop out; don't laugh, it's harder than you think. The sun is shining, and it is a great feeling. I'm thinking, *Free at last, free at last, thank God Almighty, I am free at last.* I remember watching the news on August 28, 1963, when CBS broadcasted Martin Luther King Jr.'s "I Have a Dream" speech.

However, my freedom is cut short when my eighty-five-pound, all-muscle Bernese mountain dog, Matilda, charges toward me. As is her routine, she leaps up and pushes her paws against my chest, forcing me into my new car, which sets off the car alarm. Great to be back home, no joke.

I head for the garage and survey the various gas canisters, regulators, hoses, and fittings, wondering how I'll manage all of this. Then, I spot the Chock full o'Nuts coffee can—the very thing that got me into this situation in the first place. The one they used back in 1966 for the *9 Evenings* at the Armory show to make the snowflakes rise.

I pick it up and talk to the can: "We're going to do this thing for Harold, as well as just for the hell of it."

Talking to a can? Ha, maybe they released me prematurely.

The *Silver Pillows*, Warhol's favorite creative piece of "art," is in excellent shape. I inflate one with the nitrogen/helium combo, carry it to the living room, and watch it float in midair—"Neat," as Harold would say.

My balls should be finished in a week or two, at most. Lovely Wife reminds me that Keith has completed the *Marilyn Monroe* exhibit, and the Marilyn Monroe dresses and wigs are here. In the meantime, she has been studying that scene from *The Seven Year Itch* to get the look right. Lovely Wife is even channeling Marilyn by walking around the house in a blond wig—no complaints from me.

Now I just have to persuade Brad to finish the *Rising Snowflakes* project, specifically tricking out two more Chock full o'Nuts cans so the nitrogen-helium mixture will flow through the soapy water, creating the magical rising column of bubbles. The concept is similar to the child's toy where you dip a plastic ridged hoop into a bottle of soapy water, forming a film of soap on the hoop, then hold it up to your mouth and blow. A stream of bubbles flows from the hoop, and kids giggle joyfully as they chase and pop the bubbles. However, it's become apparent that solving the *Rising Snowflakes* puzzle won't be child's play. I'm wiped out and head for bed.

The next morning, I skip Brad and head to Day Camp, which, as expected, sucks—with one surprising exception. Let me start with the suck part. I have a poor sense of direction, as I may have mentioned earlier. On my first day, I spend half an hour just trying to locate the right parking lot and building. Every day at Day Camp, I'm handed a schedule. The first task is to check into the computer room where I have to take the same online test every day. It poses the usual questions, including several iterations of my favorite, "Have you had thoughts of harming yourself?" I finish this quickly, in just a couple of minutes. However, things spiral downhill from there, as I just can't figure out the schedule. The schedule lists the classes for each day of the week. Each day's schedule is different. There are five sets of columns, one each for Monday, Tuesday, and so on, side by side. Each day has three sub columns: the time of the class, the room number, and the name of the class.

The problem is that the columns are arranged contrary to the way a normal human would do it. Bafflingly, the class topic is listed first, followed by the room number, and then the time. Any sensible schedule would list the time first, class topic second, and room third. I'm starting on a Tuesday, which makes it even more confusing. As a result, I'm always off by a day; I attend Wednesday's classes on Tuesday, and so on. It's a disaster. They take attendance, and when my name isn't called, they point me to the door. To make things worse, I am so drugged up that I misplace my schedule at least once a day and often need to visit the office and ask for a replacement. Sometimes they become agitated, which makes me hesitant to approach them.

The medical director contacts Lovely Wife, expressing concern about my memory issues. The staff has observed me wandering the hallways or heading to the cafeteria, skipping class altogether. He wonders if I have a learning disability. Lovely Wife informs him that I am a high-functioning individual, and if I appear otherwise, it's probably due to the excessive medication they're giving me.

I attend a grand total of just two of the sixty classes over the course of two weeks. The first one starts out with the teacher forgetting to take attendance. Instead, he begins by asking each of us to share our traumatic experiences with the class, suggesting that it might aid in the healing process. I'm thinking, *Do I really belong here?*

There is some really bad stuff, really, really bad stuff that is revealed; I won't go into the details. Finally, it's my turn, and I describe my exasperating experience with Dr. Ratched.

Barely thirty seconds in, the teacher jumps up, exclaiming, "You don't belong here. This class is for patients who have suffered severe trauma."

I'm thinking, *But she did traumatize me*, followed by, *That's what he gets for being lazy and not taking roll call like all the other teachers.*

He finishes with a flourish, "GET OUT."

The second class, titled Anger Management, is insightful, and, surprisingly, I'm supposed to be here. I do have anger issues. I get angry at stupid people and situations caused by stupid people, and most people are stupid. The nugget that's revealed: NAT. For those unfamiliar with anger management lingo, NAT stands for negative automatic thought. The name says it all. Some of us are predisposed to find flaws and focus on the negative without even realizing it. I love it; I am so guilty of this.

I must admit when I first encountered the acronym NAT, I thought it was stupid. Why didn't the idiots who came up with it call it a ghastly negative automatic thought, or GNAT? Gnats are pesky insects to be avoided at all costs. Additionally, they overlooked another potential aphorism by Eldridge Cleaver, a member of the Black Panther Party, in 1968: “The price of hating someone else is loving yourself less.” This could shorten to “Hate less, love yourself more,” or HaLeLoYoMo. That would have been a much better acronym. Nonetheless, the concept of NAT doesn’t suck, and I sometimes use it to annoy others.

So it goes, a daily trip to Brad, who fiddles and diddles but doesn’t complete the *Rising Snowflakes* project, just goes through the motions. On these visits, I try not to have any GNATs. After all, Brad is a “kindred spirit” and the only one who can do the job. I’m confident he will come through in the end. Bipolars do best when up against a deadline; Brad will bring out his inner Hulk.

CHAPTER 18

"LOVELY WIFE'S 'THIRTY-NINTH' BIRTHDAY CELEBRATION"

TWO WEEKS LATER

On my final day, the medical director calls me into his office. He's not pleased with my outpatient experience. I quickly agree, assuring him we are on the same page there. He's not sure if I'm prepared to depart without additional support.

I laugh and ask, "How many of your outpatients have a job waiting for them?"

That's a rhetorical question. I'm fairly certain the answer is none, except for one, me.

I continue, "My board of directors is eager for my return. I appreciate your concern, but at this point, resuming my normal schedule is the best therapy."

He signs my discharge papers, hands them to me, and I exit. I take the papers and decide to skip the day's classes—after all, who would notice?—and head for my Tesla to drive home.

Lovely Wife is surprised that I'm returning so early.

I tell her, "They let me go on good behavior."

Arriving unannounced is always a gamble; you can fill in the rest of this thought yourself. I tell her to ignore me and go about her usual routine. Today, I have to concentrate on finalizing the venue for our grand event.

We require a venue that can host over a hundred attendees and offers convenient access for limos transporting us from the primary event in Chelsea to the after-party at GB's SoHo gallery.

The space also needs a high ceiling to accommodate the rising snowflake columns of bubbles that can reach heights of twenty-five feet or more, and an area for the silver clouds to drift freely. It must have excellent acoustics for the opera singers, Emmett, and Kerin—they may be my friends, but no doubt, they are a divo and diva, respectively. Additionally, there should be a dedicated spot for the Marilyn Subway Grate exhibit, with a dressing area, and finally, a place for the bar.

I reach out to GB to see if he and Jack, the gallery manager, can show me the space they have arranged for the show.

He responds, "Come on down tomorrow. Can you be here at 11:00 a.m.? You can buy me lunch."

"I'm there," I tell him.

For the record, some say GB has "alligator arms" when it comes to picking up the lunch tab. I believe they warrant a more artsy description: *Venus de Milo* arms.

I head off for New York City at 7:00 a.m. This is the first day in a while that I haven't visited Brad, but I told him yesterday that I wouldn't bug him for a few days—not that it would make a difference anyway. I did arrange for us to meet up this Sunday afternoon, his one half-day off. I proposed that we work on the project and not stop until it's done. He muttered a terse "Yeah." I also suggested he drive his vintage Mercedes so we could ride around South Boston, top down.

Once on the Mass Pike, I plug "GB Gallery, SoHo" into the GPS and tune to the Simon & Garfunkel streaming channel on the radio. "Mrs. Robinson," from the movie *The Graduate*, is playing. Did I mention I love that song? I must have. I make it down in about three hours and thirty-five minutes, which is pretty good considering I stop to recharge at the Hamden, Connecticut, Tesla Supercharging station, which takes about fifteen minutes.

I find free parking on Thompson Street, just a two-minute walk to the gallery.

GB greets me with his customary “Great to see you.”

I reply, “Likewise.”

Don’t think for a second that this banter is genuine—just our polite repartee, concealing the witty jabs we keep to ourselves.

We set out for lunch right away; we’ll talk business afterward. Jack stays behind at the gallery, busy with preparations for an upcoming show. Since I’m footing the bill for lunch, I suggest the falafel place around the corner, the Ba’al Café. It boasts a 4.5 rating on Yelp from 311 reviews, and just one $. The falafels, as usual, do not disappoint, and come to a total of $23.15 for three, with one for Jack.

On the way back, GB mentions he’s compiling a guest list for the event. I inform him that I’ll have fifteen to twenty guests. GB assures me he’ll populate the rest of the list with high-value attendees: art critics, collectors, art journalists, business tycoons, and supermodels. GB explains that the latter are always a big draw.

Entering the gallery, I spot Jack in the middle of a large crate. I resist the wisecrack, “Jack in the box.” Okay, I confess—remember, I am clinically unfiltered—so I say it. Jack isn’t as amused as I. He pops out of the box, and we head to the event space in Chelsea by Uber.

Upon our arrival, so far so good. The venue is on Twenty-Third Street in Chelsea, a two-way crosstown street with plenty of limo access and several nearby subways for the thrifty. We head upstairs, not a good sign as second floors are sometimes second choice. We enter a room, and it is . . . perfect. Large enough for our expected crowd, featuring tall ceilings with vaulted skylights suitable for *Rising Snowflakes* and a side area perfect for the *Marilyn’s Dress* exhibition. Finally, there’s a staged area for the opera singers, one of those spaces designed for photo shoots of models, complete with two tall walls with a rounded corner, even a spot for the piano. It’s a huge relief—the space ticks all the boxes. GB and Jack did a great job.

As I’m leaving, GB casually remarks, “I’ll see you in a couple of days.”

It takes a moment to register, but then it hits me: Lovely Wife’s birthday is in TWO days! To refresh your memory, this all began when I tried to merge Lovely Wife’s surprise celebration of her thirty-ninth birthday with the big *Defying Gravity* show. That decision ultimately landed me in Summer Camp, necessitating the separation of the two events.

I immediately call my daughter. Thankfully, she has everything under control for Lovely Wife's September 5 birthday extravaganza. My only responsibility is to show up at Bobo on West 10th with her and inform the greeter about our 7:30 p.m. reservation.

Next on my list is a call to Paul. He informs me of an issue with the base of the cradle: The curve on the top of the railroad track renders it unstable. He wants me to come in tomorrow morning to review his solution, reassuring me with, "Don't worry. I have something that should work."

While I really wanted to incorporate the tracks as a nod to Newton and Einstein, I concede my manic enthusiasm may have gotten the worst of me. Mania is like that: When you are flying high, you believe that your idea has unparalleled brilliance, and when you come back down to earth, you wonder, *What the hell was I thinking*? I'm sure Paul's solution will be just fine.

Paul is an early bird, arriving at the workshop at 5:00 a.m. every day, even though the shop doesn't officially open until 7:00 a.m. He uses the quiet time to prepare for the day's work. I arrive at 5:30 a.m. and notice the cradle sitting on the railroad tracks. Paul nudges the cradle; it rocks. The cradle is not supposed to rock.

Paul apologizes, "I tried everything, even flipping the rails upside down, but the rounded part—where the train wheels go—was unstable either way. I even tried to level off the rounded part with a grinder, but railroad tracks are extremely hard. They're made of carbon steel, and it just busted the grinder."

I look around and find his proposed replacement lying on the floor: an I-beam. Ah, the I-beam. First patented by the Belgian company Forges de la Providence in 1849, it revolutionized construction, enabling buildings to be erected taller and more quickly.

Their secret? An I-shape can resist bending and twisting better than any other form. For my purposes, its industrial, rugged look perfectly complements the smooth, polished, rounded surfaces of the stainless-steel frame. It will indeed work.

I assure him, “No problem. The I-beam will look great.”

He points over to the side of the shop where an I-beam lies: “We’ve got plenty in stock.”

I can tell he’s pleased with the substitute; he is beaming. This gives him legitimate pride of ownership of a part of *Newton’s Balls*. The good news is that Paul and Zach have figured out how to attach the wires seamlessly into both the balls and cradle. It’s an engineering marvel. I give Paul a hug, a double thumbs-up, and bid him . . . adieu. I don’t bother seeing Brad the gas guy; I’ll focus on him later. He’s the last piece of the puzzle, or possibly the last straw.

There’s no need to check in with Keith, the Marilyn Monroe subway grate guy. He seems to have everything under control. I’ll touch base with him after I return from New York City. Oh yeah, New York City. Today is September 4. Lovely Wife’s birthday is tomorrow night, and we have a lot to do.

I call my daughter, and she says, “Everything is set. I’ve been to the restaurant, and it’s perfect. Emmett is bringing his pianist, and there’s a good spot for him to play.”

I think, *He’s got his own pianist? I guess that’s what makes a divo* a *divo.*

Now comes the tough part: informing Lovely Wife of a last-minute change in plans. She’s expecting to leave for New York City tomorrow, on her birthday. She usually needs at least a week’s notice before she can adjust her plans. I, on the other hand, can zig and zag with little notice. So, I employ a self-fulfilling prophesy on her—I tell her something that will be true but isn’t quite true when I say it.

“A while ago, your mother called. She wanted to take you out for your ‘big’ birthday. I messed up and forgot about it until now. She’ll be really disappointed. Maybe we can go down to Connecticut, and she can take us out to dinner tonight. Afterward, we could head to SoHo.”

Lovely Wife is not pleased, but shockingly, she has already picked out an outfit for tomorrow night, along with a spare. Her makeup kit is always packed, and she knows a place in SoHo to have her nails done properly. Most crucially, there’s a Drybar right next to the SIXTY SoHo Hotel, where we are staying. Not familiar with Drybar? It’s for blowouts.

Next, I need to turn my little untruth into the truth. I call Babs, her mother, and let her know we are taking her out to dinner tonight to celebrate her Lovely Daughter's big birthday. She simply asks when we are picking her up, and mentions she wants to pay. Babs is much more flexible than Lovely Daughter. We set the time for 6:00 p.m. at her favorite restaurant, the Red Rooster, in Wilton, Connecticut. Dinner goes well. We drop Babs off and head to SoHo.

We check into our room at SIXTY SoHo. Lovely Wife unpacks her bags. She always unpacks her BAGS, plural, even for a one-night stand. As for me, I never unpack. I only bring what I'll wear. We eat on the walk back to the hotel and turn in early.

In the morning, I stop by Ground Support on West Broadway for an espresso. I drink it there, then order a short, quadruple shot, bone-dry cappuccino, made with skim milk, in a double cup to keep it hot—very hot. Getting this right is crucial. If I mess it up, the day can't be salvaged.

I give Lovely Wife a call: "I just received a text canceling our reservation at the Blue Ribbon Brasserie due to a kitchen fire. However, I managed to snag a last-minute spot at the uber-trendy Bobo restaurant."

I spend the afternoon walking about SoHo, giving Lovely Wife room to groom.

We meet up at the hotel, and hop into our preordered black Suburban SUV Uber—only the best for Lovely Wife on her big birthday—and arrive at Bobo on time. I give our name to the receptionist, who escorts us upstairs. As we reach the top, the inimitable Emmett, henceforth dubbed Hunkasaurus Rex, delivers a rendition of "Happy Birthday to You" that could only be rivaled by Marilyn Monroe's ode to JFK for his forty-fifth birthday in 1962. Jackie wasn't amused, but I thought this was pretty funny. When he finishes, she runs over and gives Emmett a hug that's a little too tight and a kiss that lingers a little too long.

Our daughter gets the well-deserved credit for pulling this off. Since Bobo serves only hors d'œuvres, at 8:30 p.m., we depart for our romantic dinner and . . . the Blue Ribbon Brasserie. I order the fried chicken, of course. She opts for her usual, the branzino.

The next morning, we head back to Boston, and it's time for me to wrap up the preparations for the show. Things are more or less under control, except for the *Rising Snowflakes* exhibit, which remains elusive. To my credit, we are trying to replicate something Genius Weird Harold did fifty-two years ago, not a trivial task. On the plus side, Harold and his daughter did provide us with one working prototype, but we need to make two more. It will be up to my eccentric genius, Brad, to pull it off—which he finally does—and mutters, "I had it figured out a while ago. I just had too much other stuff to do."

Now I have all the pieces. The event space will be available three hours ahead of the actual show—it's a tight schedule, so we have to make this work like clockwork. Paul will bring the deconstructed *Newton's Balls* from Boston, where he and Zach will reconstruct it in the SoHo gallery. Keith is bringing the disassembled *Marilyn Monroe's Dress* exhibit to the Chelsea venue, where he will assemble it again. Lovely Wife is bringing the Marilyn wigs and dresses, along with makeup and other primping apparatus.

As for me, I will handle the *Rising Snowflakes* and *Silver Pillows* exhibits. The gallery manager, Jack, who can bench press more than three hundred pounds, is in charge of the heavy lifting—literally. He's volunteered to lug the gas canisters up the stairs to the second floor of the event space; he says he can manage two at a time, one on each shoulder. The singers will handle themselves.

Lastly, GB, the gallery owner, will be the master of ceremony, hobnobbing with the art-world big shots and ensuring that his supermodel friends flirt with the biggest shots. George Wayne, the notorious former *Vanity Fair* columnist, is expected to wow the crowd with his outrageous outfit and rapier wit.

On to the show. Miraculously, everything does go like clockwork, which is entirely apropos since this event is in honor of Weird Harold, a former precision clockmaker. "Apropos?" From the French phrase from the 1660s *à propos*, meaning "to the purpose," with the emphasis on the last syllable.

The show begins in Chelsea at 6:00 p.m., prompt. Harold and his daughter arrive early and settle on a sofa in the corner by the *Silver Clouds*. He is the supernova of the show; everyone will be drawn to him. I hadn't noticed his distinctive look before.

His pants and shirt are 1960s techie nerd attire, complete with cardigan sweater—named after James Brudenell, Seventh Earl of Cardigan, who led the Charge of the Light Brigade during the Crimean War on October 25, 1854. But I'm drawn to his colorful blind man's cane, which he's holding in his left hand like a golf club. His head is tilted, eyes closed, sporting a wide squinting smile; some might call it a "shit-eating grin."

During the first half hour, guests arrive in a steady stream. They walk over to Harold and pay their respects, then mingle, chat, and drink. GB has certainly delivered; the attendees are the who's who of the art world: critics, artists, collectors, and the requisite models. I forget, did I mention the models? However, many guests are not fully appreciating the *Silver Clouds*. They walk past the objects floating in midair, without recognizing the phenomenon of homeostasis in action.

Sometimes, magic is right in front of people but goes unnoticed until it is revealed.

Borrowing GB's P. T. Barnum hat, I begin to spread the word: The *Silver Clouds* are the featured exhibit at the Warhol Museum in Pittsburgh. Warhol declared them his favorite piece in the museum, perhaps his favorite thing period—aside from his wigs. And it was Harold Hodges, the "Weird Harold" sitting on the sofa next to the clouds, who made it all happen. The next time they visit the museum and marvel at the showcased *Silver Clouds*, they will read the plaque that states "Made by Harold Hodges."

Just as I had hoped, the word spreads, and everyone begins to stare at the clouds in silence. Their expressions are filled with awe, reminiscent of humans sighting aliens for the first time in Steven Spielberg's *Close Encounters of the Third Kind*. If you're wondering what the "Third Kind" refers to, it signifies an actual alien sighting by a human.

The spotlight then shifts to the *Marilyn Monroe* exhibit, overseen by Lovely Wife. This masterpiece has guests lined up ten deep, waiting to don the blond wig, white dress, lipstick, and most importantly, the boobs: fake, but spectacular. First in line are Lovely Wife and me, and it is quite literally a blast.

The crowd is really into this, maybe a tad too much. The most enthusiastic of the group become known as the "grate grinders" and have to be pulled off. Many say it is a life-changing and life-affirming moment. Some even line up for an encore performance.

Last but not least, the self-proclaimed "Darlinka of Manhattan," George Wayne, the guy who whipped it out in front of a gang in Newark. Surprisingly, he is of partial Scottish heritage—and clad in a kilt. As some of you might know, kilt-wearers often go commando, so this will be interesting. George Wayne, it turns out, *is* going commando, but places his large hands discreetly on the family jewels, prompting gasps and resounding applause. I give him a double thumbs-up, maybe even three.

Now that the crowd is warmed up—perhaps a tad too warm—the opera singers begin their set. First a duet, "O Sole Mio," which translates to "My Sunshine," followed by Kerin's solos: "Près des Remparts de Seville" from *Carmen* and "Don't Rain on My Parade" from *Funny Girl*. Emmett wraps it up with his signature, "Figaro" from Mozart's *The Marriage of Figaro*. He bows and points to Kerin, who joins him with a curtsy.

After the applause and catcalls die down, Lovely Wife hustles over to give Emmett a hug that's again a little too tight and a kiss that lingers a little too long. It's déjà vu all over again, as Yogi Berra aptly said. My only appropriate response: Give Kerin the same treatment.

As the crowd descends on Kerin and Emmett, I get to work on the raison d'être for this whole event, the *Rising Snowflakes*. I knew this exhibit wasn't going to be a showstopper for most attendees, but I'm doing this for Harold, his daughter, and myself. I pour the soap solution into the three Chock full o'Nuts cans, each fitted with the requisite apparatus. I connect the nitrogen and helium tanks to a mixer valve and pump the gas through the tubing into each of the cans.

Slowly but surely, the columns of bubbles begin to rise. At this point, Harold stands up with his cane and makes his way to the table and begins to smile. As he had told me earlier, just because he's blind doesn't mean he can't "see." He reaches out to feel the bubbles, bends down to smell them, leans in to hear them, and finally sticks his tongue out to taste them.

He simply says, "Cool."

Mission accomplished.

A column of bubbles is rising from each of the three Chock full o'Nuts cans. This is indeed pretty cool, with the lights in the room reflecting off the bubbles in an explosion of rainbow colors. However, it is not the long, continuous, snakelike column that Harold had described in the *9 Evenings* at the Armory, which he felt compelled to have me replicate.

As things wind down, the property manager turns off the air-conditioning system, which had been causing a draft. Serendipitously, this turns out to be the missing piece of the *Rising Snowflakes* puzzle. The now still air allows the column of bubbles to rise slowly all the way the ceiling. The remaining stragglers are transfixed, declaring the sight to be amazing, even life-affirming.

"How the hell did you do that?" someone asks.

At this point, I notice a videographer is lying on his back, just below and to the side of the cans, capturing the spectacle as it unfolds. I'd forgotten that I'd planned to make a short documentary titled *Weird Harold* and had hired a young, brilliant math genius from Harvard, who also happened to be filmmaker, for the task. He tells me he's quite proficient at digital animation and plans to render an image of Harold inside one of the bubbles as it rises.

He smiles and says, "Now I know how the film ends."

The final act of the show unfolds in GB's eponymous gallery. There, we'll continue the celebration with more food and drink, and the unveiling of the world's largest well-hung balls, my *Newton's Balls*. We all line up to be limoed from the Chelsea site to SoHo. You might assume that "limoed" could be a legitimate verb; however, according to my go-to source, *Urban Dictionary*, it refers to getting "Bill Clintoned" in the back seat of a limo. I'll leave it there.

Lovely Wife and I, along with an art critic who fortuitously hopped into our limo, get out at the GB Gallery. In the front window, we see the balls in motion.

The critic exclaims, "That's incredible! I adored my Newton's cradle as a kid; this takes it to another level. It makes Jeff Koons seem passé. Who the hell made that? It belongs in the Whitney Museum."

I direct him to Paul and Zach, saying, "It's a collaborative work. Two of the artists are standing next to it now. Go speak with them."

I quickly go over to Paul and Zach and tell them to play dumb about the third member of the *Newton's Balls* team.

I explain, “Remaining anonymous will create intrigue, and besides, it’s more fun to stay invisible.”

They joke, “We’re good at dumb.”

They had skipped the first act of the show to fine-tune and polish the balls. They are so shiny that you can see your exact reflection from across the room, in all five balls, even while they’re in motion. The sound they make when they collide, *thunk, thunk, thunk*, along with the vibrations emanating from the impacts, reverberates to your core.

Across the gallery I spot GB standing next to Kerin and Emmett, our diva and divo. Unsurprisingly, Lovely Wife is also cozying up to Emmett, perhaps a little too closely, making sure his drink is properly topped off with perhaps a little too much enthusiasm. I suggest to Paul and Zach that we gather for a group photo of the gang.

As we make our way over, I get a text from Harold’s daughter. She says that Harold is exhausted, in a good way, and they are heading back to their room at SIXTY SoHo.

I relay this to the group: “Harold won’t be joining us, but he encouraged us to party like Warhol—and Harold actually did party with Warhol.”

We raise our glasses, and I toast, “To Harold, the man who defied gravity, and flew high.”

GB then lifts his glass and tips it toward me as he adds, “And to Anonymous, whose well-hung balls brought us back to earth.”

I then silently toast, “To a crazy life, and Lovely Wife.” One last time.

Still crazy after all these years
Oh, still crazy
Still crazy
Still crazy after all these years

“Still Crazy After All These Years,”
Paul Simon, 1976

The End

AFTERWORD

ALVARO PASCUAL-LEONE, MD, PHD
PROFESSOR OF NEUROLOGY,
HARVARD MEDICAL SCHOOL

This book is a moving and deeply personal account of *one* patient's experience with a potentially devastating brain disorder. And in offering us this completely subjective account, it becomes an invaluable narrative. There are no illnesses, only patients. Therefore, only a patient's perspective offers a true account of the reality of disease. It may not be the full truth, because other individual perspectives may differ, but it is true. Descriptions of the "average" or "typical" experience of a given disease are the ones that are not true, for they offer simplistic, cartoonlike representations of what many might experience when afflicted, but in fact no one ever does.

The individual perspective offered in this book is a poignant argument about why neuropsychiatry must fully transition from a disease-centered model to an individualized, precision-based approach. Treatments must be tailored not just to relieve symptom but also to preserve the person's individuality, function, capacity, purpose, and sense of self. Diagnostic categories are just labels. This requires not just changes in the practice of medicine but also in clinical research.

For too long, medicine has emphasized disease categorization and standardized treatment approaches: If a diagnosis is established, then the treatment is dictated by a given protocol, and the support for that comes from randomized clinical trials. Randomized controlled clinical trials are considered successful when the treatment protocol shows superior effect on symptoms than a sham control intervention in a population of patients randomly assigned to the intervention or the placebo groups. However, this framework is increasingly challenged by the diversity of clinical presentations among patients sharing the same diagnosis, and the diversity becomes even greater when individual circumstances—psychological, cultural, educational, social, and other factors—are considered. The results simply show whether a treatment might work better at the population level than a placebo but fail to really inform or predict the efficacy for an individual. Furthermore, the metrics of efficacy are typically the exact same ones for all patients and fail to consider each patient's priorities (i.e., "patient-centered outcomes").

Each person experiences illness in their unique, individual way, influenced by their genetics, environment and circumstances, psychology, education and upbringing, and cultural and social context. What is debilitating for one is irrelevant for another. Patient-centered care thus challenges the strict "biomedical model," which focuses on the physical and pathological processes of disease. Instead, it favors a "biopsychosocial model" that incorporates individual choice, empowers patients to define their priorities, considers the experience of illness, and seeks healing and well-being rather than symptomatic treatment or even cure of disease. "Humanistic medicine" should do that. Growing tendencies in health care speak of "personalized medicine" and "holistic or integrative medicine" to emphasize the importance of genetics, biomarkers, lifestyle, and social determinants, along with individual backgrounds, circumstances, purpose, goals, and attitudes.

The late Oliver Sacks (1933–2015) was a very articulate and determined advocate of the need to understand patients as whole persons rather than reducing them to their neurological diagnoses. In his book *An Anthropologist on Mars* (1995), Dr. Sacks tells the story of Ray, a talented jazz drummer who had Tourette's syndrome, a neuropsychiatric disease characterized by involuntary motor tics, vocalizations, and compulsive behaviors. Treatment with the antipsychotic medication haloperidol was highly effective in suppressing his tics, and his neurological exam "normalized." However, Ray hated it because he lost his creativity, energy, and rhythm, the very traits he considered integral to his musical gifts. In Ray's case, his Tourette's syndrome enhanced his abilities as a drummer. "Successful" treatment of the disease caused him to lose his rhythmic spontaneity and creative edge, and his drumming became slower, less fluid, and uninspired. It also caused him to lose his identity and sense of purpose. Sometimes, treating the disease, even successfully controlling the symptoms, comes at the cost of personal identity.

Brain diseases are not just disorders that need to be treated, controlled, or eradicated. Brain diseases can shape who we are and help define our identity. Ray decided not to take the treatment for his Tourette's syndrome, for he felt "healthier," more his true self, with the untreated disease. In fact, a vast literature suggests that brain diseases, damage, or injuries are not inherently negative but can, in fact, promote, enhance, or even *be* the cause of human talent. *The Paradoxical Brain* (2011), edited by Narinder Kapur, is a systematic exploration of this topic. The book covers research in neuropsychology, neurology, psychiatry, and cognitive neuroscience to challenge the conventional view of brain injury as purely destructive and to illustrate how brain damage or dysfunction can sometimes lead to unexpected cognitive or behavioral enhancements and gains.

John Elder Robison, in his best-selling memoir *Look Me in the Eye* (2007), reflects on his life with undiagnosed autism spectrum disorder. Gifted with unique talents, including extraordinary mechanical intuition, he was able to repair and improve cars and electronic devices far beyond typical capability, to build special-effects guitars for the rock band Kiss, and to engineer video games and toys. When he was forty, the diagnosis of autism spectrum disorder profoundly reshaped his understanding of himself and his social identity. Sometimes, getting a diagnosis changes our mindset and brings new challenges, even though the disease was there already.

In 2008 John participated in an experimental transcranial magnetic brain stimulation study at the Berenson-Allen Center for Noninvasive Brain Stimulation, which I founded and directed at Beth Israel Deaconess Medical Center in Boston. He was in part motivated by his interest to understand the impact of the disease on his brain and in part to control some symptoms. In his book *Switched On* (2016), John recounts his participation in the study and the transformative but bittersweet experience of the profound effects the noninvasive brain intervention had on his emotional world.

From a purely scientific point of view, the brain stimulation intervention confirmed the study hypotheses and led to a heightened social and emotional awareness that we expected to be transient and short-lived. John, like other study participants, experienced emotions more vividly and was able to understand emotional nuances in music, faces, and social interactions in ways he had never before. It was as if the stimulation had "turned on a switch" that allowed him to see aspects of human emotion he had previously "been blind to." However, in John's case, it caused him to also become acutely aware of past rejections, failures, and misunderstandings; it caused regret and distress; and it changed, and sometimes ruined, important personal relationships.

The transient effect of the stimulation led to a lasting process of transformation with deep existential consequences that, as scientists, we had not anticipated. His story is not only a first-person perspective of the enormous potential of neuroscience and neurotechnology but is also a cautionary tale about the personal and ethical complexities of altering brain function. Such considerations are important in research, but even more critical in clinical medicine, emphasizing the importance of putting the patient in the center of all care.

Following electroconvulsive therapy (ECT) for his psychotic depression, Ernest Hemingway said about the treatment: "What's the sense of ruining my head and erasing my memory, which is my capital, and putting me out of business? It was a brilliant cure but we lost the patient." Improving the symptoms of disease caused other symptoms, and Hemingway felt it robbed him of essential aspects of his identity as a person and a writer. The message seems clear: The treatment cured the disease but killed the person.

Hemingway's experience with ECT is personal. Not every patient has the same experience with ECT, and many feel helped by it. In addition, since 1960, when Hemingway was first treated, ECT has evolved significantly, devices have changed, anesthesia is used, and memory-sparing protocols have been developed and implemented. More generally, in the past decades, we have witnessed remarkable advances in the therapy of brain diseases.

The 1990s, designated by the US Congress as the "Decade of the Brain," catalyzed an unprecedented investment in brain research and propelled our understanding of the biological underpinnings of brain and mental illness. Since then, neuroscience and neuropsychiatry have continued to evolve, shaped by rapid technological progress.

One of the most transformative advances has been the ability to image the structure and function of the brain. Structural imaging technologies now allow for the detection of subtle cortical changes, white matter abnormalities, and early signs of neurodegeneration long before clinical symptoms manifest. Advanced electroencephalography and magnetoencephalography, functional magnetic resonance imaging, and positron emission tomography enable visualization of activity in neural networks. This has generated a deeper understanding of the neural substrates of neuropsychiatric conditions. We have come to recognize these disorders as disruptions in the activity patterns or structural integrity of dynamic brain circuits.

In parallel, biomarker research has accelerated, and cerebrospinal fluid assays, plasma-based markers, electrophysiological measures, and digital biomarkers of behavior are now central to efforts aimed at early diagnosis, prognosis, and treatment response monitoring for brain diseases. Digital technology has been particularly impactful: Digital phenotyping—for example, using smartphone sensors, speech analysis, and wearable devices—enables continuous, passive monitoring of mental states, offering unprecedented opportunities for early detection and intervention. Artificial intelligence and machine learning algorithms increasingly support diagnostic processes, capable of integrating multimodal data to generate disease-specific profiles.

Large-scale genome-wide association studies have uncovered hundreds of genetic loci implicated in diseases such as schizophrenia, bipolar disorder, dementia, and major depression, revealing overlapping biological pathways across traditional diagnostic boundaries. Polygenic risk scores hold promise for stratifying patients by their susceptibility to brain illness and tailoring preventive interventions accordingly.

The pharmacological landscape has also undergone profound

transformation. Enhanced understanding of the pathophysiology of diseases is enabling the development of mechanistically specific pharmacologic agents. Aside from the discovery of novel effective compounds, pharmacogenomics has identified polymorphisms and other genetic determinants of drug metabolism so that more targeted pharmacologic regimens can be prescribed. Recognition of the role of neuroinflammation in neuropsychiatric illness has spurred trials of anti-inflammatory agents, while long-acting injectable medications can improve adherence and treatment outcomes.

At the same time, advances in neuromodulation techniques have expanded therapeutic approaches to previously treatment-resistant neuropsychiatric disorders. These include invasive approaches such as deep brain stimulation and noninvasive modalities such as repetitive transcranial magnetic stimulation, transcranial current stimulation, temporal interference stimulation, photobiostimulation, and transcranial focal ultrasound stimulation. These technologies reflect a paradigm shift from symptom management to circuit modulation, aligning interventions with the neurobiological substrates of disease.

Despite all these and many other advances, brain disorders have become the main cause of lifelong human disability, surpassing cardiovascular disease and cancer. Presently, one in two people in the world suffers a brain-related disability, either because they have a disease or because they are the primary caregiver of someone who does, or both. Direct and indirect costs of brain-related disabilities exceed 15 percent of the world's gross domestic product, more than the cost of cancer, diabetes, and chronic respiratory disease combined. Present efforts and investments translate into increases in disability, and by 2030 the number of people affected by brain-related disability is projected to more than double and account for half of the worldwide economic impact of disability. At the same time, there are negative stereotypes, prejudicial attitudes, and discriminatory behaviors directed toward individuals with neuropsychiatric disorders. Such disorders were historically seen as moral failings, supernatural afflictions, or character weaknesses rather than medical conditions. A persistent stigma remains, even though we have never known as much about the biology of brain diseases and have never had as many tools to diagnose and treat them.

What are we missing?

We are missing *the* critical point. It is not a question of treating Tourette's syndrome, autism spectrum disorders, depression, Alzheimer's disease, dementia, Parkinson's disease, psychosis, and so on. It should be about treating Ray, John Robison, Ernest Hemingway, and each unique individual who might have a given disease. That is what this book illustrates in a personal, moving, and dramatic fashion. Treating, improving, or even curing a disease does not mean the outcome is the desirable one for a given individual.

Gregorio Marañón y Posadillo (1887–1960) was a Spanish physician, scientist, historian, and prolific writer, considered one of the most brilliant Spanish intellectuals of the twentieth century. Madrid's largest hospital, the Hospital General Universitario Gregorio Marañón, is named after him. Dr. Marañón emphasized, "No hay enfermedades, solo hay enfermos." (There are no illnesses only ill individuals [patients].)

Many notable physicians have expressed similar ideas. Hippocrates of Kos (c. 460–370 BC), considered the "Father of Medicine," admonished his students that if they had to choose to learn about the disease affecting a patient or about the patient who has a disease, they should focus on the latter. And centuries later, Sir William Osler (1849–1919), who many think of as the "Father of *Modern* Medicine," emphasized, "It is much more important to know what sort of patient has a disease than what sort of disease a patient has."

Nonetheless, the *Oxford English Dictionary* defines *medicine* as "the science or practice of the diagnosis, treatment, and prevention *of disease*" and *physician* as "a person who is trained and qualified to practice medicine." Similarly, a *psychiatrist* is defined as "an expert or specialist in psychiatry," which in turn is "the branch of medicine concerned with the causes, diagnosis, treatment, and prevention of *mental illness*." And a *neurologist* is defined as "an expert or specialist in neurology," which is "the branch of medicine that deals with *diseases and disorders of the nervous system*." These definitions parallel those offered by most reference dictionaries and textbooks of medicine, psychiatry, or neurology. Unfortunately, such definitions, like the remarkable advances in neuropsychiatry since the Decade of the Brain, forget the admonishments of Marañón, Hippocrates, and Osler: *They forget the patient.*

To enable real success, neuropsychiatry research and medical practice must change.

This book highlights the risk of the "science" of medicine, which, when decoupled from the "art" of the practice of medicine, risks the dehumanization of care by failing to consider the lived experience of the individual patient. It goes at the very central tension in neuropsychiatry: Is it enough, or even appropriate, to reduce symptoms if the treatment erodes essential aspects of a person's identity and agency?

In research, we need to focus on—rather than control for—individual differences. We need to integrate patient-reported outcomes and develop and apply individual identity-based measures that might guide treatments.

In medical practice clinicians must move beyond diagnosis toward dynamic, individualized treatment plans informed by biological data, psychosocial context, and continuous monitoring. Most importantly, physicians should not be telling patients what to do. Instead, they should leverage all their knowledge and training to give each patient all the information *they* need to enable *them* to decide what is best for *them*.

Books such as the present one reminds us of the way to get there: We must listen to each individual perspective, for they are true, and nothing is more important.

PERMISSIONS

Fake It 'Til You Make It
Lyrics excerpted from "Fake It 'Til You Make It," written by Gina Tharin, © 2018.
All Rights Reserved
Used with permission of Gina Tharin

Cell Block Tango (from "Chicago")
Words by FRED EBB Music by JOHN KANDER
© 1975 (Renewed) UNICHAPPELL MUSIC INC. and KANDER & EBB, INC.
All Rights Administered by UNICHAPPELL MUSIC INC. All Rights Reserved
Used by Permission of ALFRED MUSIC

Over The Rainbow
Music by HAROLD ARLEN Lyrics by E.Y. HARBURG
© 1938 (Renewed) METRO-GOLDWYN-MAYER INC.
© 1939 (Renewed) EMI FEIST CATALOG INC.
All Rights (Excluding Print) Controlled and Administered by EMI FEIST CATALOG INC.
Exclusive Print Rights Administered by ALFRED MUSIC
All Rights Reserved
Used by Permission of ALFRED MUSIC

We Gotta Get Out Of This Place
by Barry Mann, Cynthia Weil © 1965 Dyad Music Ltd (BMI) admin. by Wixen Music Publishing, Inc. All Rights Reserved. Used by Permission

Last Dance
from THANK GOD IT'S FRIDAY
Words and Music by Paul Jabara
Copyright © 1977 EMI Blackwood Music Inc. and Olga Music Copyright Renewed
All Rights Administered by Sony Music Publishing (US) LLC, 424 Church Street, Suite 1200, Nashville, TN 37219
International Copyright Secured All Rights Reserved Reprinted by Permission of Hal Leonard LLC

Still Crazy After All These Years
Words and Music by Paul Simon
Copyright © 1974, 1975 (Renewed) Paul Simon (BMI) International Copyright Secured All Rights Reserved Used by Permission
Reprinted by Permission of Hal Leonard LLC

Coffee Break
from HOW TO SUCCEED IN BUSINESS WITHOUT REALLY TRYING
By Frank Loesser
Copyright © 1961, 1962 (Renewed) FRANK MUSIC CORP. All Rights Reserved
Reprinted by Permission of Hal Leonard LLC

Fire And Rain
Words and Music by James Taylor
Copyright © 1969 EMI Blackwood Music Inc. and Country Road Music Copyright Renewed
All Rights Administered by Sony Music Publishing (US) LLC, 424 Church Street, Suite 1200, Nashville, TN 37219
International Copyright Secured All Rights Reserved
Reprinted by Permission of Hal Leonard LLC

I Got You (**I Feel Good**)
Words and Music by James Brown Copyright © 1966 Fort Knox Music, Inc. Copyright Renewed
All Rights Administered by Round Hill Carlin LLC All Rights Reserved Used by Permission
Reprinted by Permission of Hal Leonard LLC

Love The One You're With
Words and Music by Stephen Stills Copyright © 1970 ICONIC STILLS SONGS
Copyright Renewed
All Rights Administered by UNIVERSAL MUSIC WORKS All Rights Reserved Used by Permission
Reprinted by Permission of Hal Leonard LLC

ABOUT THE AUTHOR

JaKob Williams has excelled in two seemingly diverse worlds: finance and the arts. A founding partner of a prominent investment and asset management firm in Boston, Massachusetts, Williams served in various roles over the last thirty-seven years, including chief investment officer, president, CEO, and cochair, and earned recognition as a subject of Harvard Business School and Columbia Business School case studies. Outside the structured confines of finance, Williams is an acclaimed artist whose works have been lauded for their cultural and political significance.

Esteemed critic Donald Kuspit described one of his works as "one of the most significant pieces of political art of this generation."

In his debut memoir, *Chock Full of Nuts*, Williams reveals his deeply personal journey of living with a unique mental difference—a distinct lens through which he views and interprets the world. Drawing on his experiences in modern mental health institutions and the extraordinary moments that shaped his life, including a life-altering promise made while he thought he was dying on Mount Fuji, Williams explores the challenges and triumphs of embracing individuality.

With humor, resilience, and unflinching honesty, *Chock Full of Nuts* inspires readers to see their differences as strengths and encourages a bold, unapologetic embrace of what makes us unique.